Rorschachiana 39

Rorschachiana

Journal of the International
Society for the Rorschach

Volume 39/Issues 1 & 2/2018

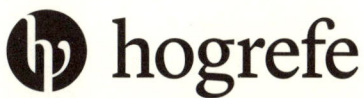

Editor-in-Chief	Sadegh Nashat, Switzerland (outgoing) / Lionel Chudzik, USA (incoming)
Advisory Editor	Anne Andronikof, France (outgoing) / Sadegh Nashat, Switzerland (incoming)
Associate Editors	Hiroshi Kuroda, Japan Justine McCarthy Woods, UK Gregory J. Meyer, USA Fernando Silberstein, Argentina
Board of Assessors	Ety Berant, Israel Sana Coderl Dobnik, Slovenia Hirono Endo, Japan Stephen Finn, USA Monica Guinzbourg de Braude, Argentina Stephen Hibbard, Canada Tuula Ilonen, Finland Sharon Rae Jenkins, USA Francis Kelly, USA Jim Kleiger, USA Joni Mihura, USA Emiliano Muzio, Finland Noriko Nakamura, Japan Daniela Nicodemo, Italy Charles Peterson, USA Vincent Quartier, Switzerland Matilde Ráez de Ramirez, Peru Pascal Roman, Switzerland Maria Concepcion Sendin Bande, Spain Bruce L. Smith, USA Jason M. Smith, USA Emine Tevfika Ikiz, Turkey Hans van Kemenade, The Netherlands Anna Elisa Villemor, Brazil Yifat Weinberg, Israel Irving Weiner, USA Latife Yazigi, Brazil
Book Review Editor	Marianne Nygren, Sweden
Editorial Assistant	Eric Ventura, Switzerland
Responsible Organization	Journal of the International Society for the Rorschach
Publication	Rorschachiana is available as a book and as a journal (consisting of two online issues per year, an annual print compendium, and online access to back issues): ISBN 978-0-88937-562-8 (Rorschachiana, Vol. 39) ISSN 1192-5604 (journal)
Copyright Information	© 2018 Hogrefe Publishing. This publication as well as the individual contributions to it are protected under international copyright law. No part of this publication may be reproduced, stored in a retrieval system, or transmitted, in any form or by any means, electronic, digital, mechanical, photocopying, microfilming or otherwise, without prior written permission from the publisher. All rights, including translation rights, are reserved.

Rorschachiana, Volume 39, 2018 (Book)

Publishing Offices	USA: Hogrefe Publishing Corporation, 7 Bulfinch Place, Suite 202, Boston, MA 02114 Phone (866) 823-4726, Fax (617) 354-6875; E-mail customerservice@hogrefe.com EUROPE: Hogrefe Publishing GmbH, Merkelstr. 3, 37085 Göttingen, Germany Phone +49 551 99950-0, Fax +49 551 99950-111; E-mail publishing@hogrefe.com
Sales and Distribution	USA: Hogrefe Publishing, Customer Services Department, 30 Amberwood Parkway, Ashland, OH 44805 Phone (800) 228-3749, Fax (419) 281-6883; E-mail customerservice@hogrefe.com UK: Hogrefe Publishing, c/o Marston Book Services Ltd., 160 Eastern Ave., Milton Park, Abingdon, OX14 4SB, UK Phone +44 1235 465577, Fax +44 1235 465556; E-mail direct.orders@marston.co.uk EUROPE: Hogrefe Publishing, Merkelstr. 3, 37085 Göttingen, Germany Phone +49 551 99950-0, Fax +49 551 99950-111; E-mail publishing@hogrefe.com
Other Offices	CANADA: Hogrefe Publishing, 660 Eglinton Ave. East, Suite 119-514, Toronto, Ontario, M4G 2K2 SWITZERLAND: Hogrefe Publishing, Länggass-Strasse 76, 3012 Bern
	Hogrefe Publishing Incorporated and registered in the Commonwealth of Massachusetts, USA, and in Göttingen, Lower Saxony, Germany Printed and bound in Germany
ISBN	978-0-88937-562-8

Rorschachiana: Journal of the International Society for the Rorschach

Publisher	Hogrefe Publishing, Merkelstr. 3, 37085 Göttingen, Germany, Tel. +49 551 999 50 0, Fax +49 551 999 50 425, publishing@hogrefe.com North America: Hogrefe Publishing, 7 Bulfinch Place, 2nd floor, Boston, MA 02114, USA, Tel. +1 (866) 823 4726, Fax +1 (617) 354 6875, customerservice@hogrefe.com
Production	Juliane Munson, Hogrefe Publishing, Merkelstr. 3, 37085 Göttingen, Germany, Tel. +49 551 999 50 422, Fax +49 551 999 50 425, production@hogrefe.com
Subscriptions	Hogrefe Publishing, Herbert-Quandt-Str. 4, 37081 Göttingen, Germany, Tel. +49 551 999 50 900, Fax +49 551 999 50 998
Advertising / Inserts	Hogrefe Publishing, Merkelstr. 3, 37085 Göttingen, Germany, Tel. +49 551 999 50 423, Fax +49 551 999 50 425, marketing@hogrefe.com
ISSN	1192-5604
Publication	Published in two online issues and a print compendium per annual volume.
Subscription Prices	Calendar year subscriptions only. Rates for 2019: Institutions - from US $259.00/€221.00 (detailed pricing can be found in the journals catalog at hgf.io/journals 2019); Individuals - US $132.00/€94.00 (print & online). Single issue (online only) - US $124.00/€97.00
Payment	Payment may be made by check, international money order, or credit card, to Hogrefe Publishing, Merkelstr. 3, 37085 Göttingen, Germany. US and Canadian subscriptions can also be ordered from Hogrefe Publishing, 7 Bulfinch Place, 2nd floor, Boston, MA 02114, USA
Electronic Full Text	The full text of *Rorschachiana* is available online at www.econtent.hogrefe.com
Abstracting Services	Abstracted/indexed in PsycINFO, PSYNDEX, Scopus, EMCare, and Cinahl Information Systems.

© 2018 Hogrefe Publishing

The Rorschach® Test has probably generated more subsequent literature in the field of psychology than any other work. Due to its universal applicability, timeless appeal to clinicians, and proven track record, this particular instrument has been utilized many millions of times throughout the world.

After 28 volumes of the Yearbook, Rorschachiana moved into a new era. Starting with the 29th volume, *Rorschachiana: Journal of the International Society for the Rorschach* has been published as a print and online journal. Subscribers to the journal have not only access to the latest research and theory on projective techniques in the two electronic online issues per year, but also to back issues, as well as online functions such as alerts, full-text searches, and many more features. In addition, *Rorschachiana* is published as an annual print compendium, in keeping with the long tradition of the Yearbook. The journal will be a useful and practical resource for experienced practitioners as well as those only beginning to develop their skills in this field.

Hermann Rorschach was born in Zurich in 1884. He studied medicine, specialized in psychiatry, and was associate director of the mental hospital in Herisau, Switzerland, when he died at the age of 37, only nine months after the publication of his now worldfamous book, *Psychodiagnostik*. Since their initial use in the early 1920s, the actual test plates have been reproduced with enormous care, to ensure that subsequent copies are precisely the same as the originals. For many decades, even the same printing presses have been used, and are maintained today exclusively for this purpose. As a result, the stimulus material has been absolutely constant for more than 80 years - a unique case in the science of psychology.

For more than 60 years, the International Society of the Rorschach and Projective Methods has played an important role in promoting the research and application of the Rorschach and other projective techniques. The first Congress of the Society took place in Zurich in August 1949. Subsequent meetings have been held periodically through the years, in a variety of locations: Rome [1956], Brussels [1958], Freiburg [1961], Paris [1965], London [1968], Zaragosa [1971], Fribourg [1977], Washington [1981], Barcelona [1984], Guarujá, São Paulo [1987], Paris [1990], Lisbon [1993], Boston [1996], Amsterdam [1999], Rome [2002], Barcelona [2005], Leuven / Louvain [2008], Tokyo [2011], Istanbul [2014], and Paris [2017]. The next meeting will be held in Switzerland in 2021.

Over these decades, ten distinguished individuals have served as presidents of the Society: Marguerite Loosli-Usteri, Robert Heiss, Adolf Friedemann, Kenowar Bash, Nina Rausch de Traubenberg, John Exner, Irving Weiner, Anne Andronikof, Bruce L. Smith, and since 2014 Noriko Nakamura.

Information regarding admission to the Society, or its various activities, can be obtained on its homepage http://www.rorschach.com or by contacting the Treasurer of the Society, Sushila Dixit, c/o Hogrefe AG, Länggass-Str. 76, 3012 Bern, Switzerland.

Contents

Volume 39, Issue 1, 2018

Research Articles	Police Trauma and Rorschach Indicators: An Exploratory Study *Tinkara Pavšič Mrevlje*	1
	Differential Performance of Professional Dancers to the Music Apperception Test and the Thematic Apperception Test *Leland van den Daele, Ashley Yates, and Sharon Rae Jenkins*	20
Original Articles	The Italian Translation of Exner's FQ Tables: Need for a Critical Edition and for a Shared Standard *Luca Angelino and Alessandra Ciliberti*	50
	SCZI or PTI – Schizophrenia or Psychosis? A Follow-Up Study *Vera Campo[†]*	76
Erratum	Correction to Vari et al., 2017 (https://doi.org/10.1027/1192-5604/a000092)	103
Obituary	Vera Campo, 1927–2018	104

Volume 39, Issue 2, 2018

Research Articles	A Normative Study in England With the Rorschach Comprehensive System *Kari Carstairs, Sarah Hartley, Andrew Peden, Justine McCarthy Woods, Andre van Graan, Anne Andronikof, and Patrick Fontan*	**105**
	Clients' TAT Interpersonal Decentering Predicts Psychotherapy Retention and Process *Sharon Rae Jenkins and Rachel B. Nowlin*	**135**
	Toward a Rorschach Hope Index *Anthony Scioli, Mike Cofrin, Friederika Aceto, and Timothy Martin*	**157**
Original Article	A Scientific Critique of Rorschach Research: Revisiting Exner's *Issues and Methods in Rorschach Research* (1995) *Jason M. Smith, Carl B. Gacono, Patrick Fontan, Enna E. Taylor, Ted B. Cunliffe, and Anne Andronikof*	**180**
Book Review	Handbook of Gender and Sexuality in Psychological Assessment *Marianne Nygren*	**204**

Research Article

Police Trauma and Rorschach Indicators
An Exploratory Study

Tinkara Pavšič Mrevlje

Faculty of Criminal Justice and Security, University of Maribor, Ljubljana, Slovenia

Abstract: This study is the first to our knowledge to focus on posttraumatic symptomatology among crime scene investigators (CSIs) and explore its relationship with their personality functioning as measured by Rorschach. Considering that posttraumatic symptomatology can affect decision-making, which is of crucial importance in police work, police officers' evaluations should include an assessment of trauma-related impairments.
The study was carried out on a sample of 64 male CSIs (85% of all Slovene CSIs). Posttraumatic symptomatology was found to be more frequent among CSIs than among the general population. Avoidance appears to be a predominant personality characteristic defending CSIs from emotionally overwhelming work situations. CSIs show less conventional, but still appropriate, cognitive mediation; however, a more detailed analysis indicates that the group with the highest posttraumatic symptomatology exhibits severely disrupted mediational processes, presumably because of negative affect.
Rorschach was found to be a suitable method for such assessments, particularly because it unfolds psychological functioning related to traumatic experience but not necessarily linked to symptoms of posttraumatic stress disorder and not necessarily recognized by the traumatized individual.

Keywords: crime scene investigators, personality, police, trauma, Rorschach

Police and Trauma

In the past few decades, the growing complexity of police tasks and the widespread application of community policing brought about a situation in which certain psychological qualities of law enforcement personnel became more important. In fact, the psychological evaluation of officers (in the selection and fitness for duty procedures; officers are referred for fitness for duty evaluation when psychological issues are assumed to be the cause of their inappropriate behavior) is indispensable for public safety. Various stress-related factors can indeed affect and impair police officers' ability to function adequately in their role and consequently pose a risk to themselves or others (Rybicki & Nutter, 2002). Police officers under stress are found to be less effective at work, experience a greater number of accidents, family violence, posttraumatic stress disorder (PTSD), depression, suicide, abuse of alcohol and illegal substances, ulcers, digestive problems, and respiratory difficulties (Marshall, 2006; Waters & Ussery, 2007). In reality, police officers are exposed to a variety of traumatic events and/or their aftermaths more frequently than is the general population (Edelmann, 2010). Therefore, posttraumatic symptomatology and PTSD among police officers are expected to a certain degree (Ballenger et al., 2010; Darensburg et al., 2006; Perez, Jones, Englert, & Sachau, 2010; Stephens & Long, 2000) and also confirmed by research (e.g., Maia et al., 2007; van Patten & Burke, 2001).

Traumatic experiences of police officers are not isolated events but rather multiple exposures (Paton, Violanti, & Schmucklet, 1999). It has been known that long-term exposures to such stressors may also evoke traumatic reactions (Herman, 1992). In fact, such symptoms may appear suddenly, intensively, and persistently, and still not meet the PTSD criteria (Marshall, 2006). Unrecognized, however, these symptoms weaken and destabilize the officer's psychological and emotional stability, which is why we prefer to use the term *posttraumatic symptomatology*.

The Use of Rorschach in Police Psychology

In the context of police psychology, psychological assessment is utilized in preemployment screenings, fitness for duty referrals, and treatment planning (Weiss, Weiss, & Gacono, 2008). The assessment of traumatic symptomatology is an important part of these evaluations. Firstly, as Buchanan, Stephens, and Long (2001) report, about 70% of police recruits have had at least one traumatic experience prior to their employment in the police force, which makes them more vulnerable for future traumatic events (Stephens, Long, & Flett, 1999). Secondly, work-related PTSD is among the most common fitness for duty referrals (Stone, 1995).

Even though Rorschach is not a predominant choice in psychological evaluations of (future) police officers (Brewster, Wickline, & Stoloff, 2010; Weiss, 2002), some of its characteristics should make it a more favorable method. One of the strongest points in this regard is its resistance to impression management in comparison with the self-reporting inventories (Weiss et al., 2008; Zacker, 1997) as the ambiguity and the absence of any clear orientation toward the "correct" answer compels the person to express genuine content (Arnon, Maoz, Gazit, & Klein, 2011). Furthermore, trauma-specific content and symptomatology are often not conscious or recognized by the traumatized individual. Nevertheless, Rorschach efficiently assesses cognitive and emotional processes affected by trauma in such cases (Sloan, Arsenault, & Hilsenroth, 2002; Tibon, Rothschild,

Appel, & Zeligman, 2011), which constitutes and additional advantage for its use in such assessments. As Weiss and colleagues conclude (2008), more research is needed to popularize Rorschach and make it more useful in police psychology. Nonetheless, it has considerable potential for application in this field.

Rorschach Trauma Assessment

The Rorschach research on trauma suffers from the same limitations as the rest of trauma research; the more sophisticated the latter, the more refined the former. Furthermore, as it is difficult to diagnose trauma by relying on clinical symptoms alone, there is no single and unique set of trauma indicators, particularly regarding the Rorschach findings (Kaser-Boyd & Evans, 2008).

Levin and Reis (1997) reviewed the literature to find common results in Rorschach protocols of traumatized people. These included higher inanimate movement responses (*m*), diffuse shading (*Y*), constricted affect or its avoidance (high *L* and low *Afr*) or unmodulated affect (unstructured color responses; *FC* < *CF* + *C*), personalized perceptions of the content of aggressive (*AG*) or morbid (*MOR*) nature influencing reality testing (*X*+%, *Xu*%, *X*−%) and interpersonal distance (*HVI*). Similar conclusions were presented by Armstrong and Kaser-Boyd (2004), who found the following common variables in traumatized clients: cognitive avoidance (high *L*, low *R*) and emotional numbing (low *Afr*, low blends), all combined in an unusually low *EB*; traumatic flooding (*CF* + *C* > *FC*); traumatic content; painful affect (high *Y* and *V*); traumatic hyper arousal (high *m* and *HVI*); and atypical views of reality (low *X*+, and high *Xu* and *WSum6*). A more recent study (Arnon et al., 2011) showed that subjects with PTSD were differentiated on the basis of 13 Rorschach indicators from the non-PTSD group: lower number of *V*, *FM*, and *T* responses; higher number of *C'* and *Cn* responses; fewer *Hh* and *Fd*, more frequent *Bt* and *Fi* answers; higher number of *INC1* responses.

Even though some common Rorschach characteristics may be found among traumatized individuals, Viglione, Towns, and Lindshield (2012) call for caution as the test may be better at describing the impact and possible forms of trauma than being a measure for PTSD.

CSIs and the Current Study

CSIs search for, collect, and analyze evidence at crime scenes. Evidence is often taken from bodies and body parts, as well as from bodily fluids, such as saliva, blood, etc. Being exposed to corpses can be particularly stressful if it happens unexpectedly and if the corpse is physically mutilated or decomposed. Moreover, such death encounters are more intense in comparison with those of other officers, since the images of death are often more graphic and violent. In addition, the search for and collection of evidence often includes examinations of decomposed bodies, and relies on sensory stimuli, such as sight, smell, and touch. Henry (2004) points out that the cumulative effect of such exposure is likely to result in long-term psychological consequences.

CSIs may be compared to other police officers with respect to the nature of their work. Nevertheless, certain characteristics mentioned earlier should be taken into account. The available literature shows that the psychological functioning and potential posttraumatic symptomatology of CSIs has been understudied (Pavšič Mrevlje, 2016). Therefore, the current study aims at exploring the potential relationships between the assessed prevalence of posttraumatic symptomatology, as measured by a self-report inventory (Detailed Assessment of Posttraumatic Stress, DAPS), and the personality characteristics of CSIs related to coping and stress management (assessed by the Rorschach test). The results presented in this paper are part of a broader study focusing on the traumatic impact on CSIs and their coping strategies.

Method

Participants

After receiving permission from the General Police Directorate, all 75 CSIs working in Slovenia at the time of this study were invited to participate. The final sample included 64 male CSIs representing 85% of the total Slovene CSI population. Five participants did not complete the Rorschach test, as they had to leave for work assignments.

The mean age of Slovene CSIs was 40.6 years ($SD = 6.97$) and 86.7% of CSIs were in a relationship. The average length of service in the role of a CSI was 12.68 years ($SD = 8.34$); however, it is difficult to report the exact number and the complexity of cases each of the participants worked on during their years of service. Nonetheless, an estimate is available for 2010 and 2011, in which a sum of 3,621 and 3,673 cases were managed, respectively (Ministry of the Interior, 2017). The average yearly workload for a CSI in these 2 years was 97.25 cases.

Measures

Posttraumatic symptomatology and PTSD were assessed by using the DAPS (Briere, 2001). The DAPS consists of 104 self-report items that are rated according to the frequency of occurrence on a 5-point scale. Apart from assessing PTSD and acute stress disorder, this instrument assesses both current and lifetime history of DSM-IV-TR trauma exposure as well as the severity and clinical significance of clients' posttraumatic symptoms, including dissociative, cognitive, and emotional responses. The DAPS also contains two validity scales that identify individuals who are under- or overreporting psychological symptoms. The DAPS – Total (PTS-T) subscale represents the total extent of respondents' PTSD symptoms and was used in the analyses presented herein.

The Rorschach test was administered to and scored by the author following Exner's Comprehensive System (CS; Exner, 1993) and considering recent CS research (Meyer, Erdberg, & Shaffer, 2007; Meyer, Shaffer, Erdberg, & Horn, 2015). To estimate the interrater reliability, 22 (37.29%) records were independently scored by another psychologist. The κ coefficients amounted to .97 for *location and space*, .88 for *determinants*, .93 for *contents*, and .80 for *special scores*, thus indicating an almost perfect interrater agreement (Landis & Koch, 1977).

The following clusters of data were included in this study: controls and stress tolerance, situationally related stress, affect, information processing, cognitive mediation (henceforth *mediation*), ideation, and Trauma Content Index (TCI; Armstrong & Loewenstein, 1990). TCI is a ratio between the sum of all blood, anatomy, sex, morbid, and aggressive movement responses and the total number of responses. It was hypothesized that a TCI of .3 or more suggests traumatic intrusions.

Procedure

The aim of this study was first introduced to the heads of all crime scene investigation departments in the Republic of Slovenia. Subsequently, individual visits to each Police Directorate were arranged between September 2010 and March 2012. The purpose of the study was presented to CSIs who were then invited to participate. Prior to the initial assessment, written informed consent was obtained. The procedures were approved by the ethics committee of the Department of Psychology, Faculty of Arts, University of Ljubljana.

The first part of the assessment (DAPS) was carried out in a group setting, while the Rorschach was applied individually. Feedback regarding individual results was offered and provided individually at a later stage.

Data were analyzed using the SPSS for Windows software (version 19.0; SPSS Inc., Chicago, IL). The Kolmogorov–Smirnov test of normality showed that data from the PTS-T scale on the DAPS were significantly different from the normal distribution ($p < .05$). Transformations of these data (log, square root, and reciprocal transformation) did not yield satisfactory results. Consequently, the Mann–Whitney test and Hochberg's GT2 post hoc test were used.

Results

The Relative Trauma Exposure as measured by the DAPS shows that the average T score is 48.04 (SD = 8.41) with a minimum of 41 and a maximum of 78. High scores on this scale indicate exposure to more events that are potentially traumatic in comparison with most people who have had at least one (Briere, 2001).

As already stated, the estimated average yearly workload of a CSI during the data collection period was 97 cases. When asked about the time of encountering their most traumatic work situation, only 51.6% replied and most of these answers (67.3%) included a case that was at least 1 year old. The participants were then asked to write about this event and 46 (75%) answered. The described cases mostly included death of an adult (60.42%) and/or death of a minor (45.83%). A smaller percentage pointed out that it was especially difficult when they had to deal with a decomposed (14.58%) and/or disfigured (10.42%) body. The remaining answers were about a direct threat to the CSI (10.42%).

The DAPS validity scales indicate an individual's tendency to deny commonly recognized symptoms (negative bias) and to over-endorse symptoms (positive bias) that are rarely endorsed by others (Briere, 2001). Negative bias was positive for 15 participants (23.4%) and positive bias for six (9.4%). The comparison between the two groups of participants (under and over the cut-off level of validity scales) on other DAPS subscales showed no significant differences (p > .05). Therefore, all participants were included in the analyses.

The PTS-T scale sums the scores of the re-experiencing, hyperarousal, and avoidance subscales. As such it reflects the total extent of PTSD symptoms endorsed by the respondent (Briere, 2001). Raw data obtained by DAPS on the PTS-T scale were converted into T scores and interpreted as follows: T scores between 60 and 65 show elevated traumatic stress that may or may not be clinically meaningful, while T scores above 65 are always clinically meaningful (Briere, 2001). As presented in Table 1, 11 participating CSIs reached the clinically significant posttraumatic symptomatology on the PTS-T scale. In addition, eight participants had elevated scores. The groups were referred to as *average*, *moderate*, and *clinical* accordingly.

The Rorschach scores are presented in Table 2. Additionally, the correlation between the TCI as a performance-based assessment and the PTS-T as a

Table 1. Crime scene investigator groups and posttraumatic symptomatology

PTS-T	f	%
Average range	45	70.3
Moderate range	8	12.5
Clinical range	11	17.2

Note. Average score on the Detailed Assessment of Posttraumatic Stress represents the average score of individuals who were exposed to at least one traumatic situation in the past. PTS-T = DAPS – Total subscale.

self-report method was computed. The results show a moderate correlation (Spearman's $r = .34$; $p = .008$).

The Mann-Whitney U test for independent samples was used to determine whether there were any statistically significant differences between the PTS-T groups regarding ideation, mediation, information processing, affect, and controls and stress tolerance. Statistically significant differences were found only in the variables related to mediation (Table 3). Hochberg's GT2 post hoc tests indicated that CSIs exhibiting clinical posttraumatic symptomatology had significantly lower $XA\%$ scores (proportion of responses with a good form fit; $p = .023$) and significantly higher $X-\%$ scores (answers that disregard reality) than the moderate symptomatology group ($p = .036$). The latter group had significantly higher $Xu\%$ scores (unusual responses) than the clinical ($p = .001$) and the average groups ($p = .012$).

Discussion

To the best of our knowledge, this is the first study investigating trauma-related phenomena in CSIs. It included 85% of Slovene CSIs (all male) in an attempt to assess the prevalence of posttraumatic symptomatology and aspects of CSIs' personality functioning linked to coping and stress management.

Clinically significant PTSD symptomatology was found in 17.2% of participants. Even though other measures should be taken into account to achieve a reliable PTSD diagnosis, the data obtained exceed the yearly prevalence of PTSD in a male nonclinical population significantly (1.8%; National Comorbidity Survey, 2005). The data of an additional 12.5% of participating CSIs who reported elevated PTSD symptomatology should also be taken into consideration. Some studies (e.g., Ozer & Weiss, 2004; Stein, Walker, Hazen, & Forde, 1997) show that individuals with elevated posttraumatic symptomatology not reaching the clinical level also suffer from symptom-related functional impairment.

Table 2. Descriptive statistics for the assessed variables on Rorschach

Variable	M	SD	Min.	Max.	Mdn
R	19.81	5.66	14.00	37.00	18.00
L	2.07	1.92	.27	14.00	1.64
EA	3.70	2.27	.00	10.50	3.00
Es	3.83	2.49	.00	11.00	3.00
Adj es	3.44	2.04	.00	9.00	3.00
EBPer	1.90	1.19	.00	3.30	2.00
D	−.03	.79	−2.00	2.00	.00
Adj D	.07	.72	−2.00	2.00	.00
FM	1.73	1.48	.00	6.00	1.00
M	.80	1.10	.00	6.00	.00
SumC'	.81	1.22	.00	7.00	.00
SumV	.03	.18	.00	1.00	.00
SumT	.08	.34	.00	2.00	.00
SumY	.37	.64	.00	2.00	.00
FC	1.07	1.00	.00	4.00	1.00
CF + C	1.10	1.08	.00	5.00	1.00
pureC	.44	.57	.00	2.00	.00
sumC'	.81	1.22	.00	7.00	.00
WSumC	1.86	1.41	.00	6.50	2.00
Afr	.50	.16	.18	.91	.50
S	1.37	1.29	.00	5.00	1.00
Blends	1.25	1.46	.00	6.00	1.00
CP	.00	.00	.00	.00	.00
A	2.93	2.32	.00	9.00	3.00
P	1.44	1.10	.00	4.00	1.00
Ma	1.02	1.34	.00	5.00	1.00
Mp	0.83	0.83	.00	3.00	1.00
2AB + Art + Ay	1.76	2.01	.00	9.00	1.00
MOR	1.22	1.59	.00	7.00	1.00
Sum6	.78	1.07	.00	5.00	.00
Lvl2	.12	.33	.00	1.00	.00
WSum6	2.56	3.91	.00	23.00	.00
M−	.15	.36	.00	1.00	.00
Mnone	.00	.00	.00	.00	.00
XA%	.83	.11	.57	1.00	.87
WDA%	.86	.11	.55	1.00	.89

(Continued on next page)

Table 2. (Continued)

Variable	M	SD	Min.	Max.	Mdn
X–%	.15	.11	.00	.41	.13
S–	.44	.68	.00	3.00	.00
P	5.08	1.82	1.00	11.00	5.00
X+%	.51	.12	.27	.79	.52
Xu%	.32	.12	.00	.61	.31
W	8.17	4.19	1.00	23.00	8.00
D	8.85	4.86	1.00	24.00	8.00
Dd	2.80	2.02	.00	9.00	3.00
M	1.52	1.32	.00	5.00	1.00
DEPI	3.47	1.16	1.00	6.00	3.00
PTI	.25	.60	.00	2.00	.00
HVI	.05	.22	.00	1.00	.00
CDI	3.46	1.04	1.00	5.00	4.00
TCI	.21	.21	.00	1.18	.17

Our results show a prominent avoidant style of the CSIs, which most likely features as a personality characteristic and less so as a defensive response style or a temporary or situational withdrawal. It appears as if this is their general way of understanding and reacting to the inner and outer triggers. Such functioning means avoiding complexity brought about by situations, relationships, and emotional experiencing (Exner, 2000). CSIs may ignore, deny, or simplify such complexity, which enables them to distance themselves from potentially overwhelming (and therefore distracting) experience, thus allowing them to focus on work tasks. Similar results were found in other Rorschach studies involving police officers (Brewster et al., 2010; Zacker, 1997), which also consider the avoidant style as limiting the impact of external stimulation, hence reducing potential overwhelming. Such functioning is helpful when working in relatively predictable and familiar crime scenes. However, it may become less effective as soon as new circumstances occur that require a more appropriate adaptation. In such instances, mental activities may become less sophisticated and emotions less effectively modulated. On the other hand, it should be noted that similar avoidant results could also be a consequence of an insufficient inquiry that may impact the Rorschach protocols, particularly the Lambda variable (Lis, Parolin, Calvo, Zennaro, & Meyer, 2007).

The reality testing of the whole group of CSIs is appropriate, but still less conventional owing to their individualistic orientation (not because of a globally

Table 3. Mediation scores for posttraumatic symptomatology

	PTS-T group	M	SD	Min.	Max.	Mdn
XA%*	Average	0.84	0.10	0.57	1	0.88
	Moderate	0.89	0.09	0.67	1	0.91
	Clinical	0.72	0.09	0.65	0.92	1
WDA%*	Average	0.87	0.10	0.55	1	0.89
	Moderate	0.89	0.11	0.63	1	0.92
	Clinical	0.76	0.09	0.68	0.95	1
X−%*	Average	0.14	0.10	0	0.41	0.13
	Moderate	0.11	0.10	0	0.33	0.09
	Clinical	0.26	0.10	0.04	0.33	0
S−*	Average	0.42	0.63	0	2	0
	Moderate	0.11	0.33	0	1	0
	Clinical	1.00	1.00	0	3	1
P	Average	5.16	1.98	1	11	5
	Moderate	4.78	1.56	2	7	5
	Clinical	5.00	1.15	3	7	5
X+%	Average	0.52	0.12	0.27	0.79	0.52
	Moderate	0.46	0.10	0.3	0.6	0.47
	Clinical	0.51	0.13	0.35	0.73	1
Xu%**	Average	0.32	0.10	0.12	0.53	0.31
	Moderate	0.43	0.10	0.27	0.61	0.43
	Clinical	0.21	0.13	0	0.38	0

Note. Statistically significant differences = Mann–Whitney U test for independent samples was used.
*$p < .05$. **$p < .01$.

disordered thought process found, for instance, in psychotic individuals). In his study of police applicants, Zacker (1997) states that unconventional interpretations could be the consequence of oversimplification linked to distorting and ignoring important features of situations. On the same note, inaccurate perceptual processes tending toward elevations in $Xu\%$ rather than $X-\%$ are characteristic of traumatized populations (Luxenberg & Levin, 2004). It is presumed that traumatic imagery disrupts thinking processes and reality testing (Ephraim, 2002 also confirms that the Rorschach documents these interferences rather well). However, this occurs only when linked to traumatic content (Viglione et al., 2012). A more detailed analysis reveals the highest level of unconventional mediation ($Xu\%$) in the moderate PTS-T group, but an even higher mediational dysfunction in the group exhibiting clinical posttraumatic symptomatology ($X-\%$). The clinical group seems to have a less appropriate understanding of their inner and outer world, as its members are likely to perceive their surroundings, other people's behavior, and themselves incorrectly. This finding is less puzzling when considering the elevated S–% responses. In fact, it is more likely that the poor judgment reflects a problem with negative affect and not a basic impairment of reality testing. This is in line with findings presented by Brewster and colleagues (2010), who report that their participating police officers showed occasionally disrupted reality testing because of feelings related to anger or hostility.

The aforementioned Rorschach indices are thus signs of traumatic functioning, particularly in cognitive avoidance, traumatically induced perceptual problems, and moderately impaired reality testing of CSIs. Similar data were also found in other Rorschach trauma studies (e.g., Armstrong & Kaser-Boyd, 2004; Luxenberg & Levin, 2004). However, these studies showed additional characteristics of traumatized individuals. Again, CSIs show posttraumatic symptomatology that impairs certain aspects of their functioning, but does not meet the criteria for a full-blown PTSD. Consequently, these investigators' difficulties may be overlooked until, unfortunately, the emergence of more prominent complications.

The TCI (= 0.21) did not reach the cut-off point of 0.3 (Armstrong & Loewenstein, 1990). As the scores of the DAPS confirm, participants had elevated but not prominent posttraumatic symptomatology, which is why a negative TCI was expected. On the same note, our study shows a moderate correlation between the TCI and PTS-T, thus supporting the findings of Mihura, Meyer, Dumitrascu, and Bombel (2013). As the authors report, there is a low correspondence between introspectively and externally assessed parallel characteristics. Moreover, in their research, Rorschach was found to complement the introspective methods – as was the DAPS used in our study. We should also consider Viglione and coworkers (2012), who argue that the TCI might be too general and miss certain unique aspects of trauma-related imagery. Perhaps the police-specific imagery could be encompassed in a specific index, similarly to the combat content score developed by Sloan, Arsenault, Hilsenroth, Harvill, and Handler (1995) for Persian Gulf War veterans.

Limitations

There are some important limitations to the present study, which need to be taken into consideration. Owing to the use of normative data instead of a comparative group, the conclusions presented by the Rorschach scores need to be interpreted prudently (e.g., Briere, 2004; Wood, Lilienfeld, Garb, & Nezworski, 2000). Additionally, despite the fact that the response rate in this study was very high, the sample size still limits its results, particularly when the sample is broken down into smaller groups for comparisons. This was a cross-sectional study, which would offer richer information about personality functioning and traumatic consequences if supported by a follow-up. Future studies should include longitudinal observations of CSIs and possibly include similar albeit other police professions, such as investigators specializing in homicides, sexual crimes, and trafficked persons. Another limitation regards the male sample of participants. Female CSIs, perhaps more common in other countries, would have shown different results.

Like other police officers, CSIs often find themselves in ambiguous, difficult, and emotionally overwhelming working situations in which they need to make clear, important, and efficient decisions. The cautiousness and avoidant functioning strategies are therefore expected or even advantageous as they enable focused mental activities in overwhelming circumstances. On the other hand, such psychological functioning may become dysfunctional and even harmful as the traumatic work experience accumulates and is not dealt with. The thin line between these two aspects is difficult to identify, as there is a broad variation in the manifestation of PTSD and posttraumatic symptomatology, which self-reporting questionnaires might overlook. Our study confirms that the Rorschach is a useful tool for describing the idiosyncratic and personal description of a person's disorder (Viglione et al., 2012) and thus recommends its use in police psychology.

References

Armstrong, J. G., & Kaser-Boyd, N. (2004). Projective assessment of psychological trauma. In M. J. Hilsenroth, D. L. Segal, & M. Hersen (Eds.), *Comprehensive handbook of psychological assessment* (Vol. 2, pp. 500–512). Hoboken, NJ: Wiley.
Armstrong, J. G., & Loewenstein, R. J. (1990). Characteristics of patients with multiple personality and Dissociative disorders on psychological testing. *The Journal of Nervous and Mental Disease, 178*(7), 448–454.
Arnon, Z., Maoz, G., Gazit, T., & Klein, E. (2011). Rorschach indicators of PTSD. *Rorschachiana, 32*(1), 5–26. https://doi.org/10.1027/1192-5604/a000013
Ballenger, J. F., Best, S. R., Metzler, T. J., Wasserman, D. A., Mohr, D. C., Liberman, A., ... Marmar, C. R. (2010). Patterns and predictors of alcohol use in male and female urban police officers. *The American Journal on Addictions, 20*(1), 21–29. https://doi.org/10.1111/j.1521-0391.2010.00092.x
Brewster, J., Wickline, P. W., & Stoloff, M. L. (2010). Using the Rorschach Comprehensive System in police psychology. In P. A. Weiss (Ed.), *Personality assessment in police psychology: A 21st century perspective* (pp. 188–226). Springfield, IL: Charles C. Thomas.
Briere, J. N. (2001). *Detailed assessment of post-traumatic stress (DAPS)*. Odessa, FL: Psychological Assessment Resources.

Briere, J. N. (2004). *Psychological assessment of adult posttraumatic states: Phenomenology, diagnosis, and measurement* (2nd ed.). Washington, DC: American Psychological Association.

Buchanan, G., Stephens, C., & Long, N. (2001). Traumatic experiences of new recruits and serving police. *The Australasian Journal of Disaster and Trauma Studies*. Retrieved from http://www.massey.ac.nz/~trauma/issues/2001-2/buchanan.htm

Darensburg, T., Andrew, M. E., Hartley, T. A., Burchfiel, C. M., Fekedulegn, D., & Violanti, J. M. (2006). Gender and age differences in posttraumatic stress disorder and depression among buffalo police officers. *Traumatology, 12*(3), 220–228. https://doi.org/10.1177/1534765606296271

Edelmann, R. J. (2010). Exposure to child abuse images as part of one's work: Possible psychological implications. *Journal of Forensic Psychiatry & Psychology, 21*(4), 481–489.

Ephraim, D. (2002). Rorschach trauma assessment of survivors of torture and state violence. *Rorschachiana, 25*(1), 58–76. https://doi.org/10.1027/1192-5604.25.1.58

Exner, J. E. (1993). *The Rorschach: A comprehensive system: V. 1: Basic foundations and principles of interpretation* (3rd ed.). New York, NY: Wiley.

Exner, J. E. (2000). *A primer for Rorschach interpretation*. Asheville, NC: Rorschach Workshops.

Henry, V. E. (2004). *Death work: Police, trauma, and the psychology of survival*. Oxford, UK: Oxford University Press.

Herman, J. L. L. (1992). *Trauma and recovery: The aftermath of violence – from domestic abuse to political terror*. New York, NY: Basic Books.

Kaser-Boyd, N., & Evans, F. B. (2008). Rorschach assessment of psychological trauma. In C. B. Gacono & B. Evans (Eds.), *The handbook of forensic Rorschach assessment* (pp. 255–277). London, UK: Routledge.

Landis, J. R., & Koch, G. G. (1977). The measurement of observer agreement for categorical data. *Biometrics, 33*(1), 159–174.

Levin, P., & Reis, B. (1997). Use of the Rorschach in assessing trauma. In J. P. Wilson & T. M. Keane (Eds.), *Assessing psychological trauma and PTSD* (pp. 529–543). New York, NY: Guilford Press.

Lis, A., Parolin, L., Calvo, V., Zennaro, A., & Meyer, G. (2007). The impact of administration and inquiry on Rorschach Comprehensive System protocols in a national reference sample. *Journal of Personality Assessment, 89*(1), 193–200. https://doi.org/10.1080/00223890701583614

Luxenberg, T., & Levin, P. (2004). The role of the Rorschach in the assessment and treatment of trauma. In J. P. Wilson & T. M. Keane (Eds.), *Assessing psychological trauma and PTSD* (2nd ed., pp. 190–225). New York, NY: The Guilford Press.

Maia, D. B., Marmar, C. R., Metzler, T., Nóbrega, A., Berger, W., Mendlowicz, M. V., ... Figueira, I. (2007). Post-traumatic stress symptoms in an elite unit of Brazilian police officers: Prevalence and impact on psychosocial functioning and on physical and mental health. *Journal of Affective Disorders, 97*(1–3), 241–245. https://doi.org/10.1016/j.jad.2006.06.004

Marshall, E. K. (2006). Cumulative career traumatic stress (CCTS): A pilot study of traumatic stress in law enforcement. *Journal of Police and Criminal Psychology, 21*(1), 62–71. https://doi.org/10.1007/BF02849503

Meyer, G. J., Erdberg, P., & Shaffer, T. W. (2007). Toward international normative reference data for the Comprehensive System. *Journal of Personality Assessment, 89*(1), 201–216. https://doi.org/10.1080/00223890701629342

Meyer, G. J., Shaffer, T. W., Erdberg, P., & Horn, S. L. (2015). Addressing issues in the development and use of the Composite International Reference Values as Rorschach norms for adults. *Journal of Personality Assessment, 97*(4), 330–347. https://doi.org/10.1080/00223891.2014.961603

Mihura, J. L., Meyer, G. J., Dumitrascu, N., & Bombel, G. (2013). The validity of individual Rorschach variables: Systematic reviews and meta-analyses of the comprehensive system. *Psychological Bulletin, 139*(3), 548–605. https://doi.org/10.1037/a0029406

Ministry of the Interior, Republic of Slovenia (2017). *Statistical data of cases investigated by the CSI.* Unpublished data, Ministry of Interior, Republic of Slovenia, Slovene Police, Ljubljana, Slovenia.

National Comorbidity Survey (2005). *NCS-R appendix tables: Table 1. Lifetime prevalence of DSM-IV/WMH-CIDI disorders by sex and cohort. Table 2. Twelve-month prevalence of DSM-IV/WMH-CIDI disorders by sex and cohort..* Retrieved from http://www.hcp.med.harvard.edu/ncs/publications.php

Ozer, E. J., & Weiss, D. S. (2004). Who develops Posttraumatic stress disorder? *Current Directions in Psychological Science, 13*(4), 169–172. https://doi.org/10.1111/j.0963-7214.2004.00300.x

Paton, D., Violanti, J., & Schmucklet, E. (1999). Chronic exposure to risk and trauma: Addiction and separation issues in police officers. In J. M. Violanti & D. Paton (Eds.), *Police trauma: Psychological aftermath of civilian combat* (pp. 37–53). Springfield, IL: Charles C. Thomas.

Pavšič Mrevlje, T. (2016). Coping with work-related traumatic situations among crime scene technicians. *Stress & Health, 32*(4), 374–382. https://doi.org/10.1002/smi.2631

Perez, L. M., Jones, J., Englert, D. R., & Sachau, D. (2010). Secondary traumatic stress and burnout among law enforcement investigators exposed to disturbing media images. *Journal of Police and Criminal Psychology, 25*(2), 113–124. https://doi.org/10.1007/s11896-010-9066-7

Rybicki, D. J., & Nutter, R. A. (2002). Employment-related psychological evaluations: Risk management concerns and current practices. *Journal of Police and Criminal Psychology, 17*(2), 18–31. https://doi.org/10.1007/BF02807112

Sloan, P., Arsenault, L., & Hilsenroth, M. (2002). Use of the Rorschach in the assessment of war-related stress in military personnel. *Rorschachiana, 25*(1), 86–122. https://doi.org/10.1027/1192-5604.25.1.86

Sloan, P., Arsenault, L., Hilsenroth, M., Harvill, L., & Handler, L. (1995). Rorschach measures of posttraumatic stress in Persian Gulf War veterans. *Journal of Personality Assessment, 64*(3), 397–414. https://doi.org/10.1207/s15327752jpa6403_1

Stein, M. B., Walker, J. R., Hazen, A. L., & Forde, D. R. (1997). Full and partial posttraumatic stress disorder: Findings from a community survey. *American Journal of Psychiatry, 154*(8), 1114–1119. https://doi.org/10.1176/ajp.154.8.1114

Stephens, C., & Long, N. (2000). Communication with police supervisors and peers as a buffer of work-related traumatic stress. *Journal of Organizational Behavior, 21*(4), 407–424. https://doi.org/10.1002/(SICI)1099-1379(200006)21:4<407::AID-JOB17>3.0.CO;2-N

Stephens, C., Long, N., & Flett, R. (1999). Vulnerability to psychological disorder. Previous trauma in police recruits. In J. M. Violanti & D. Paton (Eds.), *Police trauma: Psychological aftermath of civilian combat* (pp. 65–74). Springfield, IL: Charles C. Thomas.

Stone, A. V. (1995). Law enforcement psychological fitness for duty: Clinical issues. In M. I. Kurke & E. M. Scrivner (Eds.), *Police psychology into the 21st century* (pp. 109–131). Hillsdale, NJ: Erlbaum.

Tibon, S., Rothschild, L., Appel, L., & Zeligman, R. (2011). Assessing effects of national trauma on Adaptive functioning of mentally healthy adults: An exploratory Rorschach study. *Psychology, 2*(9), 953–960. https://doi.org/10.4236/psych.2011.29144

van Patten, I. T., & Burke, T. W. (2001). Critical incident stress and the child homicide investigator. *Homicide Studies, 5*(2), 131–152. https://doi.org/10.1177/1088767901005002003

Viglione, D. J., Towns, B., & Lindshield, D. (2012). Understanding and using the Rorschach Inkblot test to assess post-traumatic conditions. *Psychological Injury and Law, 5*(2), 135–144. https://doi.org/10.1007/s12207-012-9128-5

Waters, J. A., & Ussery, W. (2007). Police stress: History, contributing factors, symptoms, and interventions. *Policing: An International Journal of Police Strategies & Management, 30*(2), 169–188. https://doi.org/10.1108/13639510710753199

Weiss, P. A. (2002). Potential uses of the Rorschach in the selection of police officers. *Journal of Police and Criminal Psychology, 17*(2), 63–70. https://doi.org/10.1007/BF02807116

Weiss, P. A., Weiss, W. U., & Gacono, C. B. (2008). The use of the Rorschach in police psychology: Some preliminary thoughts. In C. B. Gacono & F. B. Evans (Eds.), *The handbook of forensic Rorschach assessment* (pp. 527–542). Mahwah, NJ: Erlbaum.

Wood, J. M., Lilienfeld, S. O., Garb, H. N., & Nezworski, M. T. (2000). The Rorschach test in clinical diagnosis: A critical review, with a backward look at Garfield (1947). *Journal of Clinical Psychology, 56*(3), 395–430.

Zacker, J. (1997). Rorschach responses of police applicants. *Psychological Reports, 80*(2), 523–528. https://doi.org/10.2466/pr0.1997.80.2.523

Received February 9, 2017
Revision received September 5, 2017
Accepted September 17, 2017
Published online May 9, 2018

Tinkara Pavšič Mrevlje
Assistant Professor
Faculty of Criminal Justice and Security
University of Maribor
Kotnikova 8
1000 Ljubljana
Slovenia
tinkara.pavsicmrevlje@fvv.uni-mb.si

Summary

Police officers' psychological evaluation is indispensable for public safety as various stress-related factors can affect their ability to function adequately. Crime scene investigators (CSIs) are police officers who collect and analyze evidence at crime scenes, often from bodies and body parts that can be physically mutilated or decomposed and as such constitute a stressful factor. The available literature shows that the psychological functioning and potential posttraumatic symptomatology of CSIs have been understudied. Therefore, the current study aims at exploring potential relationships between the assessed prevalence of posttraumatic symptomatology (measured by a self-report inventory) and the personality characteristics of CSIs related to coping and stress management (assessed by the Rorschach). Moreover, its purpose is to verify the use of Rorschach in the psychological assessment of police officers.

The study was carried out on a sample of 64 male CSIs (85% of all Slovene CSIs). Posttraumatic symptomatology was found to be more common among CSIs than in the general population. Avoidance appears to be a predominant personality characteristic defending CSIs from emotionally overwhelming work situations. CSIs show less conventional but still appropriate cognitive mediation; however, a more detailed analysis indicates that the group with the highest posttraumatic symptomatology exhibits severely disrupted mediational processes, presumably due to negative affect.

It is difficult to diagnose trauma by relying on clinical symptoms alone, since there is no single and unique set of trauma indicators. Nevertheless, review of the literature shows common results in Rorschach protocols of traumatized people. The aforementioned Rorschach indices are signs of traumatic functioning. To sum up, CSIs may ignore, deny, or simplify complexity, which enables them to distance themselves from potentially overwhelming experience and allows them to focus on work tasks.

Some limitations to the study, such as the use of normative data instead of a comparative group and a representative but still relatively small sample (particularly when broken down into smaller groups for comparisons), require prudent interpretation. Furthermore, the study is limited to male CSIs. Nevertheless, Rorschach was found to be a suitable method for assessing police officers, and as it is not a predominant choice in such evaluations, some of its characteristics should make it a more favorable method.

Povzetek

Psihološka ocena policistov je izrednega pomena za javno varnost, saj lahko različni stresni dejavniki vplivajo na njihovo delovanje. Kriminalistični tehniki so policisti, ki zbirajo in analizirajo sledi na kraju dogodka, pri čemer so pogosto v stiku s trupli v deli telesa, ki izmaličeni ali v procesu razkroja zagotovo predstavljajo stresni dejavnik. Pregled literature kaže, da so raziskave o psihološkem delovanju in morebitni posttravmatski simptomatiki pri kriminalističnih tehnikih zelo redke. Zato smo želeli z raziskavo ugotoviti potencialno povezavo med prevalenco posttravmatske simptomatike (izmerjeno s samoocenjevalnim vprašalnikom) in osebnostnimi lastnostmi, vezanimi na spoprijemanje s stresom (ocenjenimi z Rorschachovim preizkusom), pri kriminalističnih tehnikih. Dodaten namen je bil preveriti uporabnost Rorschachovega preizkusa za psihološko oceno policistov.

V raziskavi je sodelovalo 64 moških kriminalističnih tehnikov (85% vseh kriminalističnih tehnikov v Sloveniji). Pokazalo se je, da je posttravmatska simptomatika med tehniki pogostejša kot v splošni populaciji. Izogibanje je njihova izstopajoča osebnostna lastnost, ki jih ščiti pred čustveno preplavljajočimi delovnimi situacijami. Njihova kognitivna mediacija je manj konvencionalna, čeprav še vedno ustrezna, vendar pa natančnejša analiza kaže, da ima skupina tehnikov z najvišjo posttravmatsko simptomatiko hudo motene procese mediacije, najverjetneje zaradi negativnih čustev.

Travme pri različnih posameznikih ne moremo določiti preko edinstvenega sklopa znakov, zato jo je zgolj preko kliničnih simptomov težko diagnosticirati. Kljub temu pa je v literaturi zaslediti podobnosti v rezultatih travmatiziranih ljudi na Rorschachovem preizkusu. Zgoraj omenjeni rezultati Rorschachovega preizkusa kažejo na travmatiziranost kriminalističnih tehnikov. Če povzamemo; tehniki lahko zanemarjajo, zanikajo ali poenostavljajo kompleksnost situacij, kar jim omogoča distanciranje od morebitnih preplavljajočih doživljanj in s tem opravljanje delovnih nalog.

Raziskava ima nekatere omejitve, saj je bil za primerjavo uporabljen normativni in ne kontrolni vzorec, končni vzorec udeležencev pa je tudi relativno majhen (še posebej, ko ga razdelimo v manjše skupine za primerjave). Poleg tega so rezultati omejeni na tehnike moškega spola. Izsledke moramo zaradi omejitev pazljivo interpretirati, vendarle pa so rezultati pokazali, da je Rorschachov preizkus ustrezna metoda ocenjevanja policistov. Zaradi nekaterih njegovih prednosti pri ocenjevanju travmatiziranosti bi lahko postal pogostejša izbira psihologov, saj je v tovrstnih postopkih redko uporabljen.

Résumé

L'évaluation psychologique des policiers est essentielle à la sécurité publique car différents facteurs de stress peuvent affecter leur fonctionnement. Les techniciens de police scientifique recueillent et analysent les traces sur les lieux d'infractions. Ils sont souvent au contact de corps et parties de corps pouvant engendrer du stress. L'analyse bibliographique montre que peu d'études concernent le fonctionnement psychologique et les éventuels symptômes post-traumatiques de ces techniciens. Cette étude vise donc à établir un lien entre la prévalence des symptômes post-traumatiques (mesurée par un questionnaire d'auto-évaluation) et les traits de personnalité liés à la gestion du stress (évalués par le test de Rorschach) chez les techniciens de police scientifique, et à vérifier l'utilité du test de Rorschach pour évaluer les policiers.

64 techniciens hommes, représentant 85 % des techniciens de la police scientifique slovène, ont participé à l'étude. L'étude démontre que les symptômes post-traumatiques sont plus fréquents chez ces techniciens que dans la population générale. L'évitement, leur trait de personnalité distinctif, les protège contre les situations professionnelles émotionnellement envahissantes. Leur médiation cognitive est moins conventionnelle, bien que toujours appropriée, mais une analyse approfondie démontre que les processus de médiation du groupe souffrant le plus de symptômes post-traumatiques sont fortement altérés, probablement en raison d'émotions négatives.

Les traumatismes des individus ne peuvent être déterminés par un ensemble unique de signes et peuvent difficilement être diagnostiqués sur la base de symptômes cliniques. Néanmoins, les publications sur ce thème présentent des résultats au test de Rorschach similaires pour les personnes traumatisées. Les résultats précités montrent que les techniciens étudiés souffrent de traumatismes. Ils négligent, nient ou simplifient la complexité des situations pour se distancer des expériences envahissantes et assurer leurs missions professionnelles.

Les limites de l'étude sont l'échantillon normatif, et non de contrôle, utilisé pour la comparaison, et la taille relativement petite de l'échantillon final. En outre, les résultats sont limités à des techniciens de sexe masculin. En raison de ces limites, les résultats doivent être interprétés avec précaution, mais ils démontrent bien que le test de Rorschach constitue une bonne méthode d'évaluation des policiers. Les psychologues pourraient choisir plus fréquemment ce test compte tenu de certains de ses avantages pour l'évaluation des traumatismes.

Resumen

La evaluación psicológica de los agentes de policía es importantísima para la seguridad porque el estrés puede influirles. Los técnicos de investigación criminal son agentes de policía que recogen y analizan huellas, y suelen trabajar con cadáveres y partes desfiguradas o putrefactas, que pueden representar un factor de estrés. Los estudios existentes muestran que hay pocas investigaciones sobre el funcionamiento psicológico y su posible sintomática postraumática en los técnicos. Se ha querido determinar la relación entre la presencia de síntomas postraumáticos (con el cuestionario de autoevaluación), y las características personales vinculadas a lidiar con el estrés (según el test de Rorschach) en los técnicos. El objetivo fue verificar la utilidad del test en las evaluaciones psicológicas.

Participaron 64 técnicos varones (85 % de los técnicos de Eslovenia). Se ha demostrado que los síntomas postraumáticos entre los técnicos son más comunes que en la población general. La evitación es la característica destacable que los protege ante las situaciones emocionales vividas. Un análisis profundo muestra que un grupo de técnicos con alta sintomática postraumática tiene perturbaciones en las mediaciones, debido a emociones negativas.

Los traumas no pueden determinarse mediante un conjunto único de signos, lo que dificulta el diagnostico solo con los síntomas clínicos. Sin embargo, con el test de Rorschach pueden encontrarse similitudes en los resultados de personas traumatizadas. Los resultados de Rorschach indican el trauma de los técnicos. Los técnicos pueden ignorar, negar o simplificar las situaciones, distanciándoles de posibles experiencias para poder cumplir su trabajo.

El estudio presenta limitaciones, ya que para comparar se ha utilizado la muestra de control y no la final de los participantes y, además, ésta es pequeña (especialmente si se dividen los grupos para las comparaciones). Además, los resultados se limitan a los técnicos de género masculino. Debido a las limitaciones, los resultados se deben interpretar con cuidado, aunque, han mostrado que el test de Rorschach es el método más apropiado para evaluar a los agentes de policía. Gracias a sus ventajas en la evaluación del trauma, podría convertirse en la elección más común entre los psicólogos, aunque raramente se utiliza en estos procedimientos.

要約

警察官のトラウマとロールシャッハ指標

　警察官の心理学的評価は、多様なストレスと関連した要因が、彼らが適切に機能するための能力に影響を与えうるので、公衆安全のためには不可欠である。科学捜査研究員（CSIs）は事件現場において、しばしば切断されているとか腐敗しているといったストレス要因に満ちている遺体や遺体の一部分から証拠を集め、分析をする警察官である。入手可能な文献によれば、科学捜査研究員の心理学的な機能と潜在的な心仍外傷後ストレスの症候学は解明されてきている。それゆえ、本研究の目的は、心的外傷後ストレス（これは自己評価の調査票で測定される）の症状のアセスメントされた蔓延度と科学捜査研究員の対処やストレスマネージメントに関連しているパーソナリティ特性（これはロールシャッハ法でアセスメントされる）の潜在する関連性を探求することである。さらに、警察官の心理学的な評価においてロールシャッハ法の利用の有用性を確認することも目的である。

　本研究は64名の男性のCSIのサンプル（スロベニアの全CSIの85％にあたる）に実施された。一般的な標本においてよりも、CSIにおいて心的外傷後の症状はよりありふれていた。CSIを情緒的に圧倒させる仕事の状況から防衛する回避が、優勢なパーソナリティ特性のようであった。CSIはあまり固習的ではないが、適切な認知媒介機能を示していた。しかしながら、より詳しく分析をすると、もっとも心的外傷後ストレスが最も高かった群においては、重篤に崩壊した認知的媒介過程を示し、それはおそらく負の感情によるものである。

　単一のあるいは、特有の一組のトラウマの指標はないので、臨床症状だけを頼りにしてトラウマを診断することは困難である。それでもなお、文献レヴューによればトラウマを体験した人々のロールシャッハプロトコルには共通した結果があることが示されている。前述のロールシャッハ指標は心的外傷性の機能のサインである。要約すれば、CSIは無視、否認、あるいは複雑さを単純化し、それによって自分自身を潜在的に圧倒するかもしれない体験から距離をとることを可能にし、仕事の課題に彼らを集中させることを可能にする。

比較グループの代わりに標準グループを用いていること、代表的なサンプルであるがそれでもなおサンプル数が小さいこと（特に、比較のためにさらに小さい群に分割する場合などは）、といった研究の限界がこの研究成果の慎重な解釈を必要とする。さらに、本研究は男性の科学捜査研究員に限定している。それでもなお、ロールシャッハ法は警察官をアセスメントするのに適した方法であることがわかるが、ロールシャッハ法はそのような評価に優勢な選択ではないので、この方法の特性のいくつかはより好意的な方法とされるべきであろう。

Research Article

Differential Performance of Professional Dancers to the Music Apperception Test and the Thematic Apperception Test

Leland van den Daele[1], Ashley Yates[2], and Sharon Rae Jenkins[3]

[1]California Institute of Integral Studies, San Francisco, CA, USA
[2]Department of Psychiatry, New Hanover Regional Medical Center, Wilmington, NC, USA
[3]Department of Psychology, University of North Texas, Denton, TX, USA

Abstract: This project compared the relative performance of professional dancers and nondancers on the Music Apperception Test (MAT; van den Daele, 2014), then compared dancers' performance on the MAT with that on the Thematic Apperception Test (TAT; Murray, 1943). The MAT asks respondents to "tell a story to the music" in compositions written to represent basic emotions. Dancers had significantly shorter response latency and were more fluent in storytelling than a comparison group matched for gender and age. Criterion-based evaluation of dancers' narratives found narrative emotion consistent with music written to portray the emotion, with the majority integrating movement, sensation, and imagery. Approximately half the dancers were significantly more fluent on the MAT than the TAT, while the other half were significantly more fluent on the TAT than the MAT. Dancers who were more fluent on the MAT had a higher proportion of narratives that integrated movement and imagery compared with those more fluent on the TAT. The results were interpreted as consistent with differences observed in neurological studies of auditory and visual processing, educational studies of modality preference, and the cognitive style literature. The MAT provides an assessment tool to complement visually based performance tests in personality appraisal.

Keywords: dancers, cognitive style, kinesthetic empathy, Thematic Apperception Test, story-telling

In clinical use, the Rorschach Inkblot Method (RIM; Exner & Erdberg, 2005) and the Thematic Apperception Test (TAT; Morgan & Murray, 1935) have long been the dominant performance-based tests of implicit motivation and personality. The RIM requires participants to view ambiguous inkblots with the query, "What might this be?" (Exner & Erdberg, 2005). The TAT is a narrative-based test that invites participants to tell stories about a series of pictures (Morgan & Murray, 1935). The RIM, TAT, and derivative instruments have proven valuable for clinical assessment to generations of psychologists. The appeal of these instruments arises, in part, from the tests' sensitivity to individuality. This contrasts with self-report, true–false, Likert scaled, and other common paper-and-pencil tests that constrain agency and the individuality of response to restrictive response options (Jenkins, 2014).

However, both the RIM and the TAT, like most other personality tests, depend on visual stimuli. TAT instructions ask respondents to account for human relations, cognitive and emotional processes, actions, and outcomes inferred from pictures of people. By contrast, the Music Apperception Test (MAT) depends upon sound (van den Daele, 2007a). Music is heard and felt simultaneously, as vibration and as a propensity to movement. Unlike sight, one cannot avoid hearing the music. Participants hear it no matter how disagreeable or unpleasant. The continuing sensory intrusion sometimes elicits visceral feelings. Music characteristically induces mood or emotion that arouses feeling and memory linked to life experiences (Juslin & Sloboda, 2010). As the late Oliver Sacks (2010) noted, music activates attention and memory even among patients with advanced dementia. Thus, a music-based test may evoke qualitatively different responses than visually based tests.

Sound is mediated through subcortical processes, whereas vision is represented directly in the visual cortex. The processing of sound depends upon temporal rhythms external to the cortex, while vision is subject to cyclical processing that depends upon intrinsic cortical rhythms (Conway, Pisoni, & Kronenberger, 2009; Lewkowicz, 2000). The temporal characteristic of sound imposes duration as a facet of felt experience. This is different from the interpretive rendering of a static visual picture. Responding to continuing auditory stimuli calls forth adaptive response to real-time change. Therefore, a music-based test, with features of temporal regularity and variation characteristic of music, reveals how participants adapt to a flow of information.

Nevertheless, the TAT and MAT possess similar task requirements: narration of stories (Jenkins, 2014). The purpose of this study is to compare dancers' MAT performance with that of nonmusician adults, describe the main features of dancers' MAT narratives, and explore their relative fluency on the MAT and TAT. Relative fluency (verbal productivity) reflects associative ease and comfort, which bears on the sampling validity of the resulting narratives, that is, the extent to which a set of stories provides a representative sample of implicit narrative processes (Jenkins, 2017). The narratives of professional dancers to MAT compositions are relevant because dancers are trained to be sensitive to music connotation and emotion. Thus, dancers are likely to be quicker to tell stories and more verbally productive than are nondancers, and their narratives might represent their implicit narrative processes better than those of nondancers.

Individual Differences in Responsiveness to Auditory and Visual Modalities

The investigation of mental process in relation to auditory and visual stimuli has been largely limited to attention and recognition tasks. Psychological investigations of the relative role of auditory processes and vision in personality organization and behavior are rare, although the importance of the sound accompanying behavior in movies and the arts is well known (Cohen, 2001). The representation of motivation may be entirely transformed by its accompanying sound track. Among the few assessment studies of personality organization and behavior, the Multimodal Emotion Recognition Task (Bänziger, Grandjean, & Scherer, 2009) identified differences between visual and auditory stimuli for factor structures of emotion recognition. The authors describe an instrument that objectively measures emotion recognition based on actor portrayals of 10 emotions that combine visual and auditory sensory modalities (audio/video, audio only, video only, still picture). Factor analysis of the data from a large validation sample suggests two separate abilities, visual and auditory recognition, which appear largely independent of personality dispositions.

How the results of personality assessment may be dependent upon sensory modality is suggested by studies that employ functional magnetic resonance imaging (fMRI). This neurological assessment tool provides a view of blood flow to areas of the brain in real time. In the typical paradigm, fMRI participants are asked to attend to or engage in different tasks. Studies of modality effects for attention, memory, and emotion using fMRI show activation of supramodal networks along with activation of networks specific to vision or audition (Crottaz-Herbette, Anagnoson, & Menon, 2004; Zvyagintsev et al., 2013). The stimulation of a modal network is correlated with diminished activation of alternative modal networks. These findings suggest that both visual and auditory performance tests sample both common and unique associative material and pathways. Thus, the use of an auditory personality test may evoke content, emotion, and narration different from a visual personality test.

Historically, psychological assessment exploration of individual differences in preference for auditory or visual stimuli has been largely confined to special education and educational psychology (Sternberg & Zhang, 2001). Persons with different learning styles benefit from teaching approaches tailored to their preferred modality (Schmeck, 2013). Preference is linked to visual or auditory learning styles. Young children typically show preference for the auditory modality (Robinson & Sloutsky, 2004). Although studies find that preference for different modalities continues into adulthood (Wehrwein, Lujan, & DiCarlo, 2007), relative performance on otherwise similar visual versus auditory narrative tests of personality has not been studied.

Visual Versus Auditory Tests

Personality testing has been largely based on visual and print media. While auditory tests of implicit perception and motivation have long been proposed beginning with Skinner's tautophone (Rutherford, 2003), auditory tests failed to find a place in psychological assessment. The reasons for this may have been practical as well as theoretical. During the early history of psychological testing, sound equipment was heavy, awkward, and subject to mechanical failure. Verbal responses were fleeting. Recording equipment was subject to the same problems as sound equipment. By contrast, visual stimuli in the form of cards and the written word were light, inexpensive, and reliable. Tests that required auditory stimuli seemed more appropriate for the laboratory than the clinic.

The state of technology that shaped early testing no longer applies. Sound and recording equipment have been miniaturized and are light, inexpensive, and dependable. Assessment stimuli that involve sound and recording are practical and simple to administer and permit new methods of psychological assessment. Participants' response latencies, fluency, accentuation, pace, and prosody of speech may be recorded and quantified. Hesitations and changes in the pace of speech may reveal unacknowledged affect and competing narratives. Such information has application in diagnosis (Horowitz, 2012) and may prove helpful in treatment, particularly in methods such as therapeutic assessment (Finn & Tonsager, 1997) and collaborative assessment (Fischer, 2000), since recordings may be replayed to clients to evoke emotion or conflict.

Music and Emotion

A large and growing literature addresses the relation of music to emotion (Eerola & Vuoskoski, 2013; Elfenbein & Ambady, 2002; Juslin & Sloboda, 2010). Emotion bears a direct and immediate relation to music and is central to human cognition and behavior. Music selected to mirror emotion activates the same areas of the brain as do emotionally evocative pictures or sounds (Aubé, Angulo-Perkins, Peretz, Concha, & Armony, 2015). Tempo, key, and melody play a reliable role in the elicitation of mood and emotion in the experience of music. Sadness is connoted by slower music and happiness by faster music. Major keys suggest strength, determination, and domination, while minor keys suggest longing and melancholy. Rising melodic themes convey hopefulness and expectation; descending themes suggest introversion and reflection (Hunter & Schellenberg, 2010; Webster & Weir, 2005). Musical tempo, key, and theme interact in myriad ways to create new meanings (van den Daele, 2007a). Like emotion, music occurs not only "at a time" but "in time." The intensity of emotion ebbs and flows, and sometimes transmutes to different feelings or moods. Patterns of vital feeling are conveyed by varying prosody, breadth, intensity, pattern, and tempo (Cochrane, Fantini, & Scherer, 2013).

The Music Apperception Test (MAT)

The Music Apperception Test (MAT) evolved from the Music Projective Test (van den Daele, 1967) through successive refinement. During the development of the MAT, four different formats, durations, and mixes of music were explored. Common to all versions was the instruction to "tell a story to the music." Earlier versions were administered to a wide range of participants, including hospitalized schizophrenic patients, patients in psychoanalysis, and village children and adults in India (van den Daele, 2007a).

The outcome of experience with earlier formats is an instrument that represents basic emotions described in theories of emotion (de Rivera, 1977; Ekman, 2015; Izard, 1971). Brief pieces of music portray the emotions, and 30-s silent periods demarcate compositions. The music, written specifically for the MAT, is based upon templates that specify tempo, rhythm, number of voices, melodic line, consonance, and dissonance for the expression of emotions (van den Daele, 2007a). The compositions are titled: *Interest, Joy, Love, Desire, Shame, Excitement, Anger, Distress, Fear, Guilt, Terror,* and *Disgust.* For example, the MAT's musical portrayal of guilt suggests anguished self-blame (Plantinga, 2009). The felt quality of this emotion is conveyed by a slow ponderous, repetitive tempo, minor key, lower notes, melodic descent, and occasional dissonance. By contrast, joy is in a quicker tempo, major key, and is harmonious with a rising melodic line. As the MAT progresses through compositions, music becomes more atonal, arrhythmic, and strident. Thereby, the MAT functions as a stress test to evaluate how well respondents deal with increasingly cacophonous representations of affect.

Music emotion has been validated by several methods. First, doctoral students blind to composition emotion rank-ordered each of the aforementioned pieces of music on checklists of 12 terms. Second, narratives to compositions were coded for thesaurus agreement using the *Dictionary of Affect in Language* (DAL). The DAL is a computerized program that ascribes to emotion words a value for pleasantness/unpleasantness and for activity/passivity, creating a circumplex space within which an emotion may be located (Whissell, 2009). Therefore, an emotion may be pleasant, but not active, or active and not pleasant. Each emotion has its characteristic signature. MAT narratives to MAT music were factor analyzed for pleasantness and activity and compared with DAL norms. The results suggested that emotions occur in clusters in response to compositions (van den Daele, 2007a). For example, the emotion distress overlaps with suffering, pain, sorrow, anguish, grief, misery, worry, upset, bother, stress, and so on for a list of more than 100 related affective states. The light, lyrical compositions, *Interest, Love,* and *Joy*, elicited narratives that portrayed *Approach* behaviors; the descending, minor compositions, *Desire, Shame,* and *Guilt* elicited *Introspective* reflection; the martial tempo pieces, *Excitement* and *Anger* evoked *Urgent Action*; the cacophonous compositions, *Distress* and *Fear* provoked stories of *Adaptive Challenge*; and the variable and irregular compositions, *Terror* and *Disgust*, induced apocalyptic *Limits Testing* themes. The qualitative evaluation of narratives to individual compositions yielded empirical consistencies for hedonic tone, affects expressed, interaction, themes, and settings for each composition (van den Daele, 2007b).

Clinically, the MAT is employed along with other tests for assessment of psychological dynamics, diagnosis, and treatment planning. The test serves as an ice breaker to put clients at ease and observe the client's response to a novel situation. van den Daele (2007a, 2014) summarized clinical interpretation of the MAT and provided an example of case formulation of an individual's psychodynamics. Depending on the referral question, Response Latency may gauge quickness or impulsivity; Fluency, ease or inhibition; Narrative Style, associative or methodical thought; and Affective Fit, connection to emotion and empathy. Music that portrays emotion that is troubling for a client calls forth longer latencies, story revisions, digressions, self-critical remarks, and off-topic comments. This permits identification of emotional issues and associated defenses.

Music and Dancers

Reynolds and Reason (2012, p. 1) argued that "kinesthetic empathy" linked to music and movement transcends language and cultural differences. From a cross-cultural perspective, music, movement, and emotion are intimately related. Computer programs that transform music into visual displays of movement communicate basic emotions to viewers. To test this hypothesis, Sievers, Polansky, Casey, and Wheatley (2013) used a computer program to generate matching examples of music and movement that varied movement rate, jitter (regularity of rate), direction, step size, and dissonance/visual spikiness. The authors found that individual emotions were represented by unique combinations of features recognized both by participants in the United States and participants in an isolated Cambodian village.

Music has a natural kinship with dance. Professional dancers bear an intense relation to music and feeling expressed through movement. They engage in an occupation that distinguishes them from persons who pursue sedentary activity and abstraction. Insofar as a person's lifestyle and interests relate to personality, professional dancers are allied to persons in performing arts and to those who by occupation or disposition cultivate or possess heightened attention to movement, music, and feeling.

The Present Studies

Just as implicit and explicit memory and motivation rely upon distinct, but overlapping, neural networks (Westen, Blagov, Harenski, Kilts, & Hamann, 2006), so do auditory and visual systems mobilize distinct pathways and association areas. Visually based performance tests alone are unlikely to assess adequately the contributions of kinesthetic and auditory experience to narrative assessment data. We explored this question in the first study through comparison of the Response Latency and Fluency of dancers to those of a matched group of nondancers to see whether the professional practice of dance, an auditory-kinesthetic activity, is related to differential quickness and fluency of MAT narratives. The second study compared the relative fluency of dancers to the MAT, a music based test, and to the TAT, a visual test. The emotional fit of dancers' narratives to compositions and their narrative style were evaluated. The differential fluency of dancers to the MAT and TAT and this differential's impact on fit and style were examined, and the dancers were interviewed to elicit their experience of the tests.

Study 1 Method

Participants

We recruited 26 professional modern dancers for the study. The sample included two coastal states: California and North Carolina. All dancers had commenced the study of dance by 12 years old; they ranged in age from 21 to 65 years, with their average age being 34.7 years. Seven participants were men, 19 were women. Of the participants, 92% had completed college or an advanced degree. About 58% were Caucasian; 11% were African American; 7% were Asian, 7% Native American, and the remainder distributed among other ethnic groups.

A comparison group of nondancers who had taken the MAT was drawn from an earlier dissertation study (Quinn, 1999) that involved 168 children, adolescents, and adults and had separate IRB approval. Among these, 56 adults met selection criteria of ranging in age from 21 to 45 years, not being professional musicians or dancers, and being free from severe emotional or psychological stress. From this subgroup, a comparison group was selected to match the dancers by age and gender. The final matched groups were each composed of six men and 17 women for a total of 23 participants in each group or 46 participants overall. Three dancers over age 45 were excluded from comparisons. The average age for the matched dancers was 31.6 years (SD = 5.7) and for the comparison group 32.3 years (SD = 5.9); the average age difference between matched participants was less than 1 year. However, average education for dancers was 16.5 years (SD = 2.0) and for the comparison group was 14.7 years (SD = 2.3). The difference in education was significant, $t(44)$ = 2.80, p =.01, d = .84. Of the selected dancers, 60% were Caucasian, 9% were African American, 9% were Asian, 9% were Native American, and the remainder distributed among other ethnic groups. In all, 74% of comparison participants were Caucasian, 9% were Hispanic, 9% Asian, and 7% identified with other groups. A chi-square test for differences in ethnicity distribution was not significant, $\chi^2(5)$ = 5.64, p = .66, although dancers spanned a larger number of ethnic categories.

Measures

Music Apperception Test (MAT; van den Daele, 2007b, 2007c)
The MAT is available in four formats: A *Standard Form* composed of 10 compositions, an *Extended Form* of 12 compositions, and two *Short Forms* of four compositions each. The Short Forms sample systematically from the major MAT music groups, and the average values for response latency and fluency are virtually equivalent to those of the Standard and Extended tests (van den Daele, 2007b). All have 30-s silent periods between compositions. Each version employs the same prerecorded instructions to "tell a story to the music" followed by a brief example from *Peter and the Wolf*. Following the example, the administrator answers any questions about the procedure, and reminds the participant to "tell a story as the music plays." Some participants find the task difficult and employ the 30-s silent period to tell or complete their stories.

The *MAT Manual* defines 37 different measures in 10 categories: *Response Latency, Fluency, Time to Termination, Pace, Content, Interaction, Off-Task Response, Voice, Narrative Style,* and *Affective Fit*. Provisional norms for Response Latency and Fluency for children, adolescents, and adults are based on 2,016 narratives from 168 individuals (Quinn, 1999; van den Daele, 2007b). Since measures for other categories had not been developed at the time of the Quinn (1999) study, Study 1 compared only Response Latency and Fluency.

Response Latency is defined as the number of seconds after a composition begins to task-relevant verbalization by the participant. Fluency is defined as the number of task-relevant words spoken in response to an MAT composition. For the MAT, Fluency is confined to narration during the composition, the 30-s silent period that follows, and, infrequently, following the silent period. MAT off-task commentary is coded as *tangential* and understood as defensive or indicative of competing associative processes. With one exception, dancers' narratives were consistently on-task.

Individuals show marked consistency of Response Latency and Fluency. The early version of the test yielded average Pearson correlations among compositions of .94 for Response Latency (reaction time) and .99 for Fluency, while test-retest reliabilities after 2 weeks were .92 for Response Latency and .96 for Fluency (van den Daele, 1967). In a benchmark study of 168 participants, the split-half reliability for Response Latency was .93 and for Fluency was .91 for adults between the ages of 18 and 45 years (Quinn, 1999; van den Daele, 2007b). Since the dancers were administered the MAT Short Form B (four compositions: *Love*, *Guilt*, *Excitement*, and *Fear*), only responses to the four compositions that comprise the MAT Short Form B were employed in comparisons. The Guttman split-half reliabilities for the MAT Short Form B were .89 for Response Latency and .91 for Fluency (van den Daele, 2007b); and in the current study, .83 for both Response Latency and Fluency.

Measures of Response Latency and Fluency differed significantly between diagnosed schizophrenic patients and controls matched for gender, age, and intelligence (van den Daele, 1967). Quick Response Latency among children was correlated with poor performance on the Matching Familiar Figures Test (Kagan, 1965), widely employed as a test of impulsivity (Quinn, 1999). In another study, MAT Response Latency and Fluency clearly distinguished Samadhi, Vipassana, and Master meditation practitioners (Copenhaver, 2010).

Procedure

Following approval by the Institutional Review Board, dancers were recruited through word of mouth and personal contact with dancers known to the second author. Data were collected at convenient, private locations over 1 year. Dancers were informed that their participation was completely voluntary with no compensation, their data were anonymous, their responses were being recorded to be transcribed for accuracy, and they had the right to stop the testing at any point for any reason. All participants were asked to complete questions regarding age, gender, race/ethnicity, dance experience, education, and relationship status. An audio recorder was set up in the administration room and the MAT Short Form

B was administered. Dancers also told stories to four TAT cards used for Study 2. The order of presentation of the MAT and TAT was counterbalanced. Half received the MAT first, and half, the TAT.

The comparison group participants were recruited using flyers distributed at a community college in the San Diego area with a reward of two movie tickets. They were advised of the purpose of the research and time requirements prior to administration of the MAT. They were assured of confidentiality and advised of the right to terminate at any time, to ask questions, and to obtain a summary of the outcome of the study on request. They completed a demographic questionnaire and the vocabulary subtest of the WAIS-R. All participants were then administered the Extended Form (12 compositions) of the MAT with a duration, including instructions, of 25 min. After completing the MAT and additional tests for emotion recognition, participants were debriefed. No participants reported a negative experience, and most described the process as enjoyable.

Study 1 Results

The subsample of dancers was nearly three times faster to respond than the comparison group, having an average Latency of 8.86 s (SD = 8.67) compared with 23.42 s (SD = 18.07). The difference is significant, $t(44)$ = 3.48, p = .001, d = 1.04 (see Table 1). Checking for possible covariates, neither age nor education were significantly correlated with Response Latency for the comparison group. However, among dancers, education was related to longer Response Latency, $r(23)$ = .42, p = .046, but age was not. Male dancers averaged 6.5 s to respond (SD = 5.74) in contrast to comparison men who averaged 16.6 s (SD = 4.29), a significant difference, $t(10)$ = 3.44, p = .006, d = 2.06. Female dancers averaged 9.5 s to respond (SD = 9.3) in contrast to the comparison women who averaged 25.8 s (SD = 20.5), a significant difference, $t(32)$ = 2.99, p = .005, d = .89. Thus, group differences were not gender-specific, and within-sample gender differences were not significant.

The selected dancers' average MAT Fluency, 107.2 words per composition (SD = 37.87), was significantly greater than for the comparison group, 68.7 words (SD = 32.54), $t(44)$= 3.69, p = .0006, d = 1.09. For the comparison group, age and education were unrelated to Fluency. Among dancers, age was associated with greater Fluency, $r(23)$ = .42, p = .046; education was not. Male dancers averaged 122.7 words per composition (SD = 33.0) and comparison men averaged 47.0 words (SD = 14.7). The difference was significant, $t(10)$ = 5.13, p = .0004, d = 2.96. Female dancers averaged 101 words per composition (SD = 34.64) and comparison females averaged 73.8 words per composition (SD = 38.9). Again,

Table 1. Percent distribution of narrative style for participants more fluent to the MAT and participants more fluent to the TAT

	Narrative Style			
	Imagistic/Kinetic	Logical	Balanced	Disorganized
MAT higher	46	13	36	5
TAT higher	60	23	8	8

Note. Percent based upon evaluation of 104 narratives, 56 for participants more fluent in response to the MAT and 48 for participants more fluent in response to the TAT. MAT = Music Apperception Test. TAT = Thematic Apperception Test.

the between-sample difference for women was significant, $t(32) = 2.21, p = .03, d = .76$, for a medium effect, whereas within-sample gender differences were not significant.

Study 1 Discussion

The finding of superior Response Latency and Fluency of dancers' narratives compared with those of nondancers is consistent with theory and research that views cognition as embodied, that is, experiencing one's body in the world gives meaning to experience (Johnson, 2013). Studies in cognitive science argue that constructs such as meaning and understanding depend upon frameworks that include schema, metaphor, metonymy, and mental imagery (Nunez, 1999). These, in turn, depend upon the nature of the human body, in particular, perceptual capacities, motor skills, and acuity of sensation. An example of how the body and its posture provide a frame for meaning is the verticality schema repeated in thousands of perceptions and activities each day such as standing upright, climbing stairs, and measuring height, which provide the foundation for the understanding of progression, growth, decline, and decay (Johnson, 2013).

Although Study 1 matched dancers with nondancers for gender and age, the dancers were more educated as well as differing in ethnicity, the latter not significantly. These differences might account for the dancers' faster Latency. However, among dancers, education was related to longer Latency, and in the comparison group, education was uncorrelated with Latency. Since education correlated with Response Latency only among dancers and not among the comparison group, and in the opposite direction to account for the former's faster Latency, differential education is an unlikely explanation for the observed difference. Since ages were comparable, age difference between groups cannot account for differences in Fluency. However, the comparison group came from a different cohort. Arguably, contemporaneous influences, such as increased Internet exposure, might account for these results. This seems improbable since increased screen time and texting seem unlikely to facilitate the spontaneous fluency characteristic of dancers. Lastly, dancers narrated to the Short Form, and the comparison group, to the Extended Form, although only responses to the same compositions were compared. However, since MAT Response Latency and Fluency is consistent across compositions, performance to a Short Form or an Extended Form should be similar. Nevertheless, the finding of superior MAT performance for professional dancers awaits replication with strict comparability of participants and method.

Study 2 Method

Participants and Procedure

The pool of 26 professional modern dancers previously described for Study 1 provided data for Study 2, a descriptive within-group comparison.

Measures

Music Apperception Test (MAT; van den Daele, 2007b)
As described for Study 1, the dancers were administered the MAT Short Form B (*Love*, *Guilt*, *Excitement*, and *Fear*). Short Form B was chosen for ease of matching with TAT cards that evoke similar emotions. Among the MAT's 37 variables, Study 2 examined Response Latency, Fluency, Narrative Style, and Affective Fit since these variables are likely to reflect differences in modality responsiveness.

The categorical variable of Narrative Style is scored in one of four categories: *Kinetic/Imagistic*, *Logical*, *Balanced*, or *Disorganized*. *Kinetic/Imagistic* responses are organized around movement, sensation, and pictures. *Logical* responses have a plot or moral with a beginning, middle, and end. *Balanced* responses include elements of both plot structure and imagery. *Disorganized* responses lack coherence; narrative perspectives are confused and story lines are disjointed (van den Daele, 2007b, pp. 54–57). During development of the MAT, seven graduate students blindly rated 15 responses for *Kinetic/Imagistic*, *Logical*, or *Balanced* response styles with intraclass correlations of .82, .83, and .81, respectively (van den Daele, 2007a). The results suggest moderate agreement among raters for evaluation of narrative styles.

For this study, Narrative Style was evaluated independently by the first two authors. The total number of narratives equaled 104 (26 × 4). Exact agreement for Narrative Style occurred for 88 out of 104 narratives (85%). Differences were reconciled through conference.

The Affective Fit of a response is evaluated for each composition by its agreement with facets of emotional expression found in typical responses. The first facet is *hedonic tone*: whether the narrative is pleasant, neutral or unpleasant. The second facet is *affect expressed* designated by a set of emotions associated with a composition. The third category is *conventional reference* subdivided into common themes, types of interactions, and settings depicted in typical responses. Only one feature of conventional reference is necessary to obtain a score of 1 – although oftentimes, narratives contain all three features. To attain the overall maximum score for Affective Fit, the narrative must be positive for the three major categories. If a narrative attains a 3, Affective Fit is *excellent*, 2 is *satisfactory*, 1 is *poor*, and 0 is *unsatisfactory*. The percent agreement among seven graduate students who blindly rated 15 responses for the *MAT Manual* was 100% (van den Daele, 2007a). In the current study, Affective Fit was independently evaluated by the first two authors. The correlation between raters for Affective Fit was .92. Again, differences were reconciled through conference to obtain exact agreement.

As an example of how to score the MAT for these categories, a dancer's response to the composition *Guilt* illustrates features of MAT narratives:

> So, this is kind of sinister and dark feeling to me, feels pretty gothic. Maybe I'm in an old European Cathedral on really cold stone floors and, um, the coldness of the stone kind of starts with the soles of my bare feet and then travels up through my body and, um, affects my movement, feels really constricted and then you know, uh, I feel that big cymbal clang or whatever that big sound is, it's almost like getting whipped or something, um, something is lurking, hiding behind the organ, it's going to come out and get me, um, so I am creeping around hiding behind the pillars of the structure not wanting to be seen or found. Yeah, I think I just really want to hide, and it's very jolting.

The narrative was voiced in the present tense. The respondent attended to realtime change, the feel of the floor, the "clang" of the gong, and "creeping around." Throughout the narrative, sensation, emotion, and movement were linked. The respondent organized her story by reference to her experience of her body. Response Latency was 4 s, Fluency 128 words, Narrative Style was predominantly Kinetic/Imagistic, and Affective Fit received a 2, indicating moderate agreement with the music's mood. In this example to *Guilt*, the respondent provides a metaphor of how guilt feels to her. Throughout the commentary, the source of affect is external but invasive, and it stirs fear, paralysis, and the desire to hide. The feeling is associated with church, gothic structures, getting whipped, and "something" lurking. She, like a child, wants to hide. As may be expected, such narratives often link to memories and central emotional conflicts.

Thematic Apperception Test (TAT; Murray, 1943)
Four TAT cards likely to elicit themes of love, guilt, excitement, and fear were selected to parallel the MAT compositions as judged by a psychologist consultant and the first two authors. Card 10, chosen to elicit love, is a close-up picture of an elderly Caucasian couple embracing, with their eyes slightly open, but not looking at each other. Card 13MF, picked to elicit guilt, depicts a woman lying on a bed with her breasts uncovered and her arm hanging limply. A man stands in front of the bed with his arm raised over his eyes. Card 17BM depicts excitement by showing a male acrobat climbing a rope. Card 15 represents fear via a graveyard setting in which a tall man in dark clothing looks down as he places his hands together and faces the ground (Murray, 1943).

TAT cards were administered in the same order to all participants. Standard TAT instructions and procedures were employed (Murray, 1943). Participants were asked, "What is happening in the picture? What happened before? How are people in the picture feeling? How are they thinking? How does everything turn out in the end?" The questions were asked in sequence, and answers recorded to each question. No additional inquiries were made. The researcher kept the cards in a pile face down, provided one card at a time, and asked the participant to place the card face down as the story was completed. The average TAT administration took about 25 min. TAT Fluency was coded as the total number of words spoken in response to the standard directions and inquiries.

Study 2 Results

In this phase of our investigation, we focused on within-group comparisons and measures of Affective Fit and Narrative Style. First, we summarized results for MAT and TAT Fluency and associations with demographic variables that may be identified as covariates. Second, we described dancers' Affective Fit of MAT responses to music compositions. Third, we examined their relative Fluency to the TAT and MAT, comparing Response Latency, Affective Fit, and Narrative Style for dancers who were more fluent on the MAT than the TAT with those who were more fluent on the TAT than the MAT. Finally, we inquired about participants' experience of the two tests. In the examination of relative responsiveness to the MAT and TAT, participants served as their own control. Therefore, a large number of nuisance variables were reduced or eliminated. However, in the interest of discovering possible confounding influences on MAT and TAT performance, we evaluated the association of gender, age, and education to these tests.

Fluency for MAT and TAT

The average word count among dancers for the MAT was 110.1 (SD = 43.1) and for the TAT was 109.7 (SD = 83.2). The difference was not significant, $t(37)$ = .03, p = .51, d = .01. Fluency to the MAT and TAT was uncorrelated, $r(25)$ = .11, p = .60. However, the standard deviation for the TAT (SD = 83.2) was nearly twice that of the MAT (SD = 43.1). The variance ratio test of difference was significant, $F(25, 25)$ = 3.72, p =.0008. When the MAT was administered first, the average fluency for the MAT was 116.77 (SD = 44.52) and for the TAT it was 113.90 (SD = 102.74), $t(15.8)$ = 0.09, p = .92. d = .01 When the TAT was administered first, the average fluency for the MAT was 103.60 (SD = 41.06) and for the TAT it was 105.46 (SD = 58.13), $t(21.1)$ = 0.09, p = .92, d = .03. The mean and SD values did not differ from one another with the exception that TAT variance was greater when the MAT was administered first, $F(12, 12)$ = 3.12, p = .03.

The individual joint variability of MAT and TAT Fluency is shown in Figure 1, with MAT Fluency ordered from low to high in relation to TAT Fluency. MAT Fluency ranged from a low of 266 words per protocol or an average of 67 words per composition to a high of 844 words per protocol or an average of 211 words per composition. TAT Fluency ranged from a low of 74 words per protocol or 19 words per card to a high of 1,492 words per protocol or 373 words per card. The order of test administration noted in the figure is unrelated to relative differences in MAT or TAT fluency.

The average MAT Fluency for male dancers was 126.9 words per composition (SD = 38.0), and for female dancers, 104.0 words per composition (SD = 43.5), although the difference was not significant, $t(11.7)$ = 1.21, p =.12, d = .56. TAT Fluency per card averaged 109.7 words (SD = 83.2). The average TAT fluency per card for male dancers was 136.5 words (SD = 127.4), and for female dancers, 99.8 words per card (SD = 57.4), a nonsignificant difference, $t(6.4)$ = 0.73, p = 0.48, d = .45. MAT Fluency was correlated with age, $r(25)$ = .47, p = .02, but not education, $r(25)$ = −.03, p = .89. TAT Fluency was marginally but nonsignificantly correlated with age, $r(25)$ = .35, p = .09, and education, $r(25)$ =.29, p = .16.

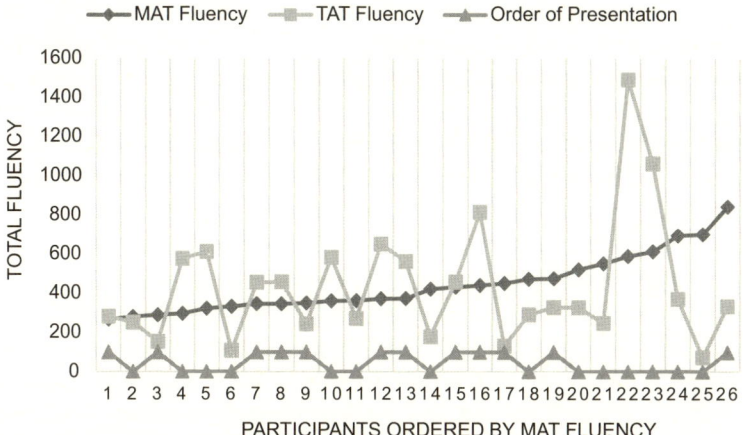

Figure 1. Total MAT Fluency from low to high and TAT Fluency by respondent. Total fluency is the sum of narrated words. 0 = MAT administered first; 100 = TAT administered first. MAT = Music Apperception Test. TAT = Thematic Apperception Test.

Affective Fit

Narratives to individual MAT compositions were evaluated for hedonic tone, expressed emotion, theme, interaction, and setting. The majority of dancers' responses (62%) obtained the maximum score for Affective Fit (AF = 3); four out of five (80%) were judged satisfactory (AF = 2) or excellent (AF = 3). Very few responses (2%) failed to meet any criteria for Affective Fit (AF = 0).

Comparing Relative MAT and TAT Fluency Groups

A slight majority of dancers (n = 14) were more fluent to the MAT than the TAT (higher MAT fluency group). For these 14 respondents, MAT Fluency averaged 117.9 words per composition (SD = 43.8), and TAT fluency per card averaged 75.4 words (SD = 55.5), 63% of the MAT Fluency. By contrast, 12 participants were more fluent on the TAT than the MAT (higher TAT fluency group). Among this group, TAT fluency per card averaged 164.7 words (SD = 81.4), and MAT Fluency per composition averaged 97.8 words (SD = 26.2), approaching half (59%) of their TAT fluency. Differences in MAT and TAT fluency were independent of the order of MAT and TAT administration. The mean age of the higher MAT fluency group (M = 34.6 years, SD = 7.7) and the higher TAT fluency group (M = 34.8 years, SD = 12.4) was similar as were other demographic characteristics.

Response Latency for the higher MAT fluency group averaged 8.37 s ($SD = 10.11$) and 9.04 s ($SD = 5.03$) for the higher TAT fluency group. Average Affective Fit for the High MAT group was 2.41 ($SD = .45$) and for the High TAT group it was 2.38 ($SD = .45$). However, participants higher in MAT Fluency more often told Balanced stories that required the integration of movement, sensation, with a story that included the development of a theme (Table 1). A test of the difference for Narrative Style between these groups was significant, $\chi^2(3) = 11.31$, $p < .02$. Cramer's V for independent groups was equal to .64 for a large effect size.

Posttest Interview

We wondered if dancers would respond to the MAT in the same way as did visual artists to the TAT who found the TAT cards poorly executed (Roe, 1946); would they be inhibited by their critical appraisal of the music? After the assessment, we asked participants how they reacted to the two tasks. All of the participants questioned, except one, stated that they "liked" the MAT better than the TAT. Reasons included the TAT was outdated; the music was exciting and ignited choreography ideas; and the TAT was "dark and depressing." Some dancers said the MAT allowed for the creation of any characters in any relation, and "I like music better than pictures." The one exception was a participant who stated he did not like the music compositions because they elicited emotions he did not want to share with the researcher in a first meeting.

Study 2 Discussion

Differences in MAT and TAT performance between higher MAT and higher TAT fluency respondents were large and noteworthy. The different characteristics of the stimuli, along with the differing instructions, necessarily create differences in the response process (Bornstein, 2007, 2011). For participants generally, responses to TAT cards were constrained by the concrete scene depicted. Dancers' responses to TAT questions focused upon the scene itself, causality, interpersonal motivations, thoughts, feelings, and dynamics. Without these visual cues, responses to MAT compositions depended upon the mood of the music, otherwise permitting free construction and elaboration of scenarios and action. Dancers' responses emphasized movement, physical sensation, emotional engagement, visualized scenes, and associative reflection. Stories often involved reminiscences and were suggestive of day-dreaming and solitary fantasy.

Within these constraints, the higher TAT fluency group was more attentive to TAT visual cues, shading, human body and facial expression, interpersonal nuance, and plot, and the higher MAT fluency group in response to MAT compositions was more sensate, emotionally engaged, expansive, and imaginative. As argued later in this paper, the tests appeared to engage different cognitive networks, but individual differences influenced responses to both visual and auditory tests. Although as shown in Study 1 dancers were generally more responsive to the MAT than were nondancers, in Study 2 dancers evidenced these individual differences and did not share a singular personality style.

The finding that the differential fluency is linked to differences in Narrative Style accords with the literature on personal style and sensory preference (Schmeck, 2013). In addition, studies of emotion recognition and the neuropsychology of sensory processing are consistent with the observed differences (Sevdalis & Keller, 2011). Results from neuropsychological investigations identify distinct visual and auditory association areas (Damoiseaux et al., 2006). The relative independence of these areas and their differential processing accord with individual differences in responsiveness and stories told to the MAT and TAT.

For narrative tasks such as the MAT and TAT, Fluency is an indicator of motivation, comfort, and openness during testing, and thus is arguably an indicator of sampling validity (Jenkins, 2017). Although the overall means of MAT and TAT Fluency did not differ, the greater individual differences for TAT Fluency suggest greater variability among dancers in sampling validity of stories told to these visual stimuli, given the lack of time constraints on TAT responses. When the MAT was administered first, the variance of TAT fluency increased. Story-telling to music may prime participant emotions that facilitate or inhibit continued story-telling.

The dancers' comments on their experiences of the two tests support the idea that differential comfort with the visual stimuli underlay their differential productivity. Examiners observed that some respondents appeared to freeze as if they were being tested when faced with a picture. Rather than stimulating the free flow of narration, the visual task appeared to inhibit their Fluency. Given that dancers achieved greater Fluency per minute with the MAT than the TAT despite the MAT's strict time limits, future research should examine whether Fluency is an independent predictor and/or an important validity indicator equally for the MAT and TAT, whether they are differentially linked to auditory versus visual system activation, and whether differential Fluency is related to differential activation. The similarity of Latency and Affective Fit between the higher MAT fluency group and the higher TAT fluency group suggest that if these groups do differ in sensory network activation, reaction speed and the implicit processing of emotion may not be centrally involved in that activation.

Molnar-Szakacs and Overy (2006) argue that music induces the activation of mirror neurons that potentiate a cascade of analogous movement and emotion. fMRI studies strongly suggest that playing or listening to music is reliably associated with activation of the frontal–parietal network (Meister et al., 2004). In turn, the frontal–parietal network is associated with autobiographical memory and directive control of conscious content (Smallwood, Brown, Baird, & Schooler, 2012). How this plays out in different narrative styles might depend on individual differences in the relative activation of cortical and subcortical sensory centers. Future research relating MAT narrative styles to activation should consider relatively high versus low TAT fluency as a possible moderator variable that identifies an important individual difference.

Dancers are oriented to movement. Movement stimulates and motivates. On the TAT, without the flow of music, some participants reported feeling distanced from their vital core and imagination. An example that illustrates the impact of MAT and TAT Fluency is a dancer's response to the composition *Love* followed by his response to the TAT card 10 (love):

> MAT (Love): So... a long time ago there was a guy named Tumefesis, and he had a very strange defect, and his penis came out of his back, and in order to keep it erect he had to talk, talk about his emotions and how he felt and, um, he became world famous as a great lover 'cause women wanted to know how he felt and he... say [sic] "oh my gosh I love being with women" so as long as they would listen, he would mate with them... so he fathered an entire kingdom called Husomondia. And, in Husomondia they grew a special kind of food that had medicine in it as so [sic] everybody was really, really healthy, and they were very, very happy and they lived in little mud houses, and they didn't wear shoes [music stops] but they wore really, really heavy gloves because all of the trees...the plants that they grew had sticklers. One of the side effects of growing this great food with medicine in it was that they were all thorny. And so they all had to wear these gloves, so that's their little story.

The dancer's Response Latency was 14 s and his Fluency was 188 words. His Affective Fit was coded 3 or excellent, and his Narrative Style was judged primarily Logical. In response to TAT card 10 (love), the same participant replied: "They're synchronized swimmers, and they were really hoping to win and they didn't, so they are consoling each other."

The MAT narrative dealt with a love theme, albeit through metaphorically inverted sexuality, patriarchy, return to nature, survival, and an elixir food/medicine. The TAT narrative, although brief, summarized need for achievement through movement, disappointment, and adaptive response. For this participant, the MAT and TAT appeared to elicit content, motives, and patterns of thought from different spheres of mental activity. The same relative differences in fluency and imagination applied to the participant's remaining MAT and TAT narratives.

Dancers more fluent on the TAT and those more fluent on the MAT did not differ from one another for Response Latency or Affective Fit. However, the higher MAT fluency dancers more often voiced a Balanced Narrative Style, 36% compared with 8% for higher TAT dancers. A Balanced narrative weaves together imagery, movement, and story line as illustrated by this response to the MAT composition *Love* from a dancer more fluent on the MAT than the TAT:

> There are trees and birds and it's a sunny day and water was flowing. And there was this beautiful Chinese dancer, and she was splaying her arms and walking gracefully down the path, and her silken fabric was flowing behind her – and it was silk and magenta and yellow. And her hair was beautiful, and anyway she was very graceful, and her hand was flowing and she started to paint. She [sic] starting to paint with her fingers, and her finger was starting to extend out, and she started to draw the clouds, and she would drag them down and then grab some more clouds and drag it down, and she starting [sic] weaving through the air and started to wisp the clouds into yarn or string, and she started to create beautiful shapes that were like spider webs, but they were glistening and dewy and the ocean was right there which was also glistening [music stops], yes, it was very lovely.

The dancer's Response Latency was 2 s and her Fluency was 163 words. Her Affective Fit was coded 3 or excellent. Movement and imagery convey nuances impossible or difficult to convey by propositional language alone.

Affective Fit requires narrative congruity with the mood or emotion conveyed by a composition. The majority of dancers' narratives scored 3 or excellent fit on a scale of 0–3. Dancers' imagery and stories were highly attuned to music nuance. This finding accords with theories and observations that connect music, movement, and emotion together (Cochrane et al., 2013). The correspondence of dancers' narrative moods to MAT music supports the content validity of the compositions for eliciting the designated emotions.

The current study found a low, but positive, correlation between dancers' ages and MAT Fluency. In previous research, age related to fluency for children. It was found that 8-10-year-old children had significantly lower Fluency to the MAT than adolescents or adults, while adolescents and adults did not differ (Quinn, 1999; van den Daele, 2007a). Greater maturity might produce greater task focus and engagement, or dancers' life experience associated with age or cohort membership might increase the contextual press to tell stories.

This study focused on general Fluency to MAT compositions and TAT cards as a proxy for associative readiness and productivity. We did not examine the effects of individual MAT compositions or TAT cards, for example, whether the MAT *Love* composition scores were correlated with or were relatively more efficacious predictors than those for a TAT love card. Similarly, the study did not address questions about the effectiveness of individual compositions or cards to instill moods or evoke mental sets. These remain questions for future research.

Finally, MAT and TAT results might have been made more comparable by adjustment of the TAT instructions to "tell a story to the picture" within an allotted time. That is, TAT instructions could have been modified to make them equivalent to the MAT. The changed procedure might have altered results to render TAT narratives higher or lower in fluency. Future research might employ more strictly comparable procedures to distinguish differential processing speed.

General Discussion and Conclusion

Dancers were significantly quicker and more fluent in verbalizing to music than were participants of the comparison group, suggesting that the music-based test may have better sampling validity (see Jenkins, 2017) for them than for nondancers. The practiced association of music and story inherent in professional dance appears to prime these participants to grasp quickly the emotional connotations of music regardless of their response to visual stimuli. The majority of dancers' narratives were embodied in a kinesthetic/imagistic or balanced narrative style. Such narratives, because they include physical sensations and actions, convey an intimacy of feeling and spontaneity. Nevertheless, dancers were about equally divided between those more fluent on the MAT and those more fluent on the TAT.

Research on the MAT is in its infancy. This is a preliminary study. The significant results are suggestive but subject to sample selection and small size, thus limited in generalizability. The instructions for the MAT and TAT are not the same. Telling a story about a TAT card with instructions that ask about the past, present, future, and the thoughts and feelings of those pictured is different from telling a story to music with less specific instructions. Instructions might have been modified for the TAT cards to simply request participants to "tell a story" about what the card depicts. This would have provided a better experimental comparison between stimuli, but would no longer entail a comparison between clinical tests. In addition, different TAT cards might have been employed to compare with music compositions. For example, although this was not a focus of the study, card 13MF has a draw for sexual themes and may not elicit guilt – although guilt, remorse, and adultery were common themes.

Despite the present intriguing findings, much remains to be done to develop the MAT's currently limited clinical utility. Thus, we end with an agenda for future studies. A first line of research related to neurological differences in auditory and visual processing (Zvyagintsev et al., 2013) would extend the present findings to examine differential fluency to auditory versus visual stimuli in the general population. Is differential fluency linked to differential validity, or to other personality or behavioral differences? Given the recent interest in storytelling from a neuroscience perspective (Finn, 2012; Mar, 2011), one potentially fruitful question concerns the pathway from perception through processing (cognitive, emotional, motivational) to physical activation and verbal expression in narrative. Are the routes through this pathway similar or different for visual versus musical stimuli? Specifically, do these routes differ for people who are differentially activated by these two stimulus classes? What if any is the role of differential fluency or other scores in stories told about pieces representing different emotions?

The story examples given in this paper suggest that the MAT not only uses a different stimulus modality for story elicitation, but also elicits qualitatively different narratives than visual TATs do. Further research is needed on the unique features of MAT narratives and the scoring categories that capture them, including those not used in this study. The MAT *Kinesthetic/Imagistic* narrative style often lacks a narrative story line and thus is much less common in stories to visual stimuli, in part because standard administration of the latter asks for a story that would score as *Logical* "with a beginning, middle, and end telling what is happening, what led up to the picture, and how it will end." Even the MAT stories told by dancers that had this logical structure often mixed in kinesthetic/imagistic elements, especially if they were more fluent to the MAT than the TAT. Whereas visual stimuli depicting people tend to draw on social cognitive theory of mind operations (Jenkins, 2017), the MAT is explicitly designed to elicit emotional operations, and these could be asocial.

Conceptual refinement is needed to frame the scoring categories, which currently rely primarily on content validity, as constructs that can be validated empirically as scores. Only a few scoring categories have been developed, and these are specific to the MAT. More scoring categories might prove useful for different storyteller populations. The generalizability of MAT scoring categories to visual TAT stories and TAT scoring categories to MAT stories merits exploration. For example, evaluation of the maturity of stories told to the MAT by measures such as the Social Cognition and Object Relations Scales (SCORS; Stein et al., 2015) may clarify the developmental role of emotion in cognition and defense.

A second, related question examines associations between MAT scoring categories and scores on conceptually related categories of other free-response measures. For example, recent research on associations between Rorschach Comprehensive System Human Movement and neurobiological mirroring activity (EEG-mu suppression; Porcelli, Giromini, Parolin, Pineda, & Viglione, 2013) is consistent with a connection between perceptions, imagined bodily activity, brain function, and verbalization. It is also consistent with our finding of a high frequency of MAT *Kinesthetic/Imagistic* narrative style in this sample of dancers. Might people who tell more *Kinesthetic/Imagistic* MAT stories have more Human Movement in their Rorschach protocols?

A more practical question concerns the ways in which human personality is shaped by life experience. The content validity of the MAT categories of *Kinesthetic/Imagistic* narrative style and *Affective Fit* suggests that future research should examine differential scores for individuals in occupations characterized by different degrees of these functions, compared with individuals not engaged in such activities. For example, hypothetically, athletes might be higher in *Kinesthetic/Imagistic* narrative style, but not *Affective Fit,* than nonathletes; musicians might be higher in *Affective Fit,* but not *Kinesthetic/Imagistic* narrative style, than nonmusicians.

Extending this reasoning into the realm of psychological disorders, do individuals with alexithymia show lower fluency on the MAT than visual TATs, or score more poorly on *Affective Fit*? Might persons with different emotional disorders tell different stories to the stimuli representing problematic versus nonproblematic emotions? Are these scores related differentially to more complex emotions represented on the MAT? Might the MAT be useful in eliciting narratives from individuals with high functioning autism or other social deficits, who might have difficulty responding to socially cued pictures? Could the combination of the MAT and visual TAT be used to identify whether a client's problems with empathy are related to deficits of social cognition versus responsiveness to emotional stimuli? Might this differential be related to the Rorschach Experience Balance (EB)? Is *Kinesthetic/Imagistic* narrative style or *Affective Fit* related to face-to-face emotional responsiveness or empathy? Addressing these questions will expand the MAT's currently limited empirical research base and begin to define its realm of clinical utility.

Acknowledgments

This paper augments and extends Yates's (2012) PsyD dissertation on modern dancers.

All participant quotes in the paper are used with participants' permission.

References

Aubé, W., Angulo-Perkins, A., Peretz, I., Concha, L., & Armony, J. L. (2015). Fear across the senses: brain responses to music, vocalizations and facial expressions. *Social Cognitive and Affective Neuroscience, 10*(3), 399–407. https://doi.org/10.1093/scan/nsu067

Bänziger, T., Grandjean, D., & Scherer, K. R. (2009). Emotion recognition from expressions in face, voice, and body: The Multimodal Emotion Recognition Test (MERT). *Emotion, 9*(5), 691–704. https://doi.org/10.1037/a0017088

Bornstein, R. F. (2007). Toward a process-based framework for classifying personality tests: Comment on Meyer and Kurtz (2006). *Journal of Personality Assessment, 89*(2), 202–207. https://doi.org/10.1080/00223890701518776

Bornstein, R. F. (2011). Toward a process-focused model of test score validity: Improving psychological assessment in science and practice. *Psychological Assessment, 23*(2), 532–544. https://doi.org/10.1037/a0022402

Cochrane, T., Fantini, B., & Scherer, K. R. (2013). *The emotional power of music: Multidisciplinary perspectives on musical arousal, expression, and social control.* New York, NY: Oxford University Press.

Cohen, A. J. (2001). Music as a source of emotion in film. In P. N. Juslin & J. A. Sloboda (Eds.), *Music and emotion: Theory and research* (pp. 249–272). New York, NY: Oxford University Press.

Conway, C. M., Pisoni, D. B., & Kronenberger, W. G. (2009). The importance of sound for cognitive sequencing abilities: The auditory scaffolding hypothesis. *Current Directions in Psychological Science, 18*(5), 275–279. https://doi.org/10.1111/j.1467-8721.2009.01651.x

Copenhaver, G. A. (2010). *Music apperception performance testing with meditation practitioners of Samadhi and Vipassana, and masters of Madhyamika.* San Francisco, CA: California Institute of Integral Studies.

Crottaz-Herbette, S., Anagnoson, R. T., & Menon, V. (2004). Modality effects in verbal working memory: Differential prefrontal and parietal responses to auditory and visual stimuli. *NeuroImage, 21*(1), 340–351. https://doi.org/10.1016/j.neuroimage.2003.09.019

Damoiseaux, J. S., Rombouts, S., Barkhof, F., Scheltens, P., Stam, C. J., Smith, S. M., & Beckmann, C. F. (2006). Consistent resting-state networks across healthy subjects. *Proceedings of the National Academy of Sciences, 103*(37), 13848–13853. https://doi.org/10.1073/pnas.0601417103

de Rivera, J. (1977). A structural theory of the emotions. *Psychological Issues, 10*(4), 1–178.

Eerola, T., & Vuoskoski, J. K. (2013). A review of music and emotion studies: Approaches, emotion models, and stimuli. *Music Perception: An Interdisciplinary Journal, 30*(3), 307–340. https://doi.org/10.1525/mp.2012.30.3.307

Ekman, P. (2015). *Darwin and facial expression: A century of research in review*. New York, NY: Malor Books.

Elfenbein, H. A., & Ambady, N. (2002). On the universality and cultural specificity of emotion recognition: A meta-analysis. *Psychological Bulletin, 128*(2), 203–235. https://doi.org/10.1037/0033-2909.128.2.203

Exner, J., & Erdberg, P. (2005). *The Rorschach, advanced interpretation*. Hoboken, NJ: John Wiley & Sons.

Finn, S. (2012). Implications of recent research in neurobiology for psychological assessment. *Journal of Personality Assessment, 94*(5), 440–449. https://doi.org/10.1080/00223891.2012.700665

Finn, S. E., & Tonsager, M. E. (1997). Information-gathering and therapeutic models of assessment: Complementary paradigms. *Psychological Assessment, 9*(4), 374–385. https://doi.org/10.1037/1040-3590.9.4.374

Fischer, C. T. (2000). Collaborative, individualized assessment. *Journal of Personality Assessment, 74*(1), 2–14. https://doi.org/10.1207/S15327752JPA740102

Horowitz, M. (2012). *States of mind: Analysis of change in psychotherapy*. New York, NY: Springer Science & Business Media.

Hunter, P. G., & Schellenberg, E. G. (2010). Music and emotion. In M. R. Jones, R. R. Fay, & A. N. Popper (Eds.), *Music perception* (pp. 129–164). New York, NY: Springer.

Izard, C. E. (1971). *The face of emotion*. East Norwalk, CT: Appleton-Century-Crofts.

Jenkins, S. R. (2014). Thematic apperceptive techniques inform a science of individuality. *Rorschachiana, 35*(2), 92–102. https://doi.org/10.1027/1192-5604/a000065

Jenkins, S. R. (2017). Not your same old story: New rules for thematic apperceptive techniques (TATs). *Journal of Personality Assessment, 99*(3), 238–253. https://doi.org/10.1080/00223891.2016.1248972

Johnson, M. (2013). *The body in the mind: The bodily basis of meaning, imagination, and reason*. Chicago, IL: University of Chicago Press.

Juslin, P. N., & Sloboda, J. A. (2010). *Handbook of music and emotion: Theory, research, applications*. New York, NY: Oxford University Press.

Kagan, J. (1965). *The matching familiar figures test*. Boston, MA: Allyn and Bacon.

Lewkowicz, D. J. (2000). The development of intersensory temporal perception: An epigenetic systems/limitations view. *Psychological Bulletin, 126*(2), 281–308. https://doi.org/10.1037/0033-2909.126.2.281

Mar, R. A. (2011). The neural bases of social cognition and story comprehension. *Annual Review of Psychology, 62*, 103–134.

Meister, I. G., Krings, T., Foltys, H., Boroojerdi, B., Müller, M., Töpper, R., & Thron, A. (2004). Playing piano in the mind – an fMRI study on music imagery and performance in pianists. *Cognitive Brain Research, 19*(3), 219–228. https://doi.org/10.1016/j.cogbrainres.2003.12.005

Molnar-Szakacs, I., & Overy, K. (2006). Music and mirror neurons: From motion to 'e'motion. *Social Cognitive and Affective Neuroscience, 1*(3), 235–241. https://doi.org/10.1093/scan/nsl029

Morgan, C. D., & Murray, H. A. (1935). A method for investigating fantasies: The thematic apperception test. *Archives of Neurology & Psychiatry, 34*(2), 289–306. https://doi.org/10.1001/archneurpsyc.1935.02250200049005

Murray, H. A. (1943). *Thematic Apperception Test*. Cambridge, MA: Harvard University Press.

Nunez, R. E. (1999). Could the future taste purple? Reclaiming mind, body and cognition. *Journal of Consciousness Studies, 6*(11–12), 41–60.

Plantinga, C. (2009). *Moving viewers: American film and the spectator's experience*. Berkeley, CA: University of California Press.
Porcelli, P., Giromini, L., Parolin, L., Pineda, J. A., & Viglione, D. J. (2013). Mirroring activity in the brain and movement determinant in the Rorschach test. *Journal of Personality Assessment, 95*(5), 444–456. https://doi.org/10.1080/00223891.2013.775136
Quinn, K. S. (1999). *Developmental responses to the Music Projective Test* (Unpublished doctoral dissertation). California School of Professional Psychology, San Diego, California
Reynolds, D., & Reason, M. (2012). *Kinesthetic empathy in creative and cultural practices*. Bristol, UK: Intellect Books.
Robinson, C. W., & Sloutsky, V. M. (2004). Auditory dominance and its change in the course of development. *Child Development, 75*(5), 1387–1401. https://doi.org/10.1111/j.1467-8624.2004.00747.x
Roe, A. (1946). The personality of artists. *Educational and Psychological Measurement, 6*, 401–408. https://doi.org/10.1177/001316444600600309
Rutherford, A. (2003). B. F. Skinner and the Auditory Inkblot: The rise and fall of the Verbal Summator as a projective technique. *History of Psychology, 6*(4), 362–378. https://doi.org/10.1037/1093-4510.6.4.362
Sacks, O. (2010). *Musicophilia: Tales of music and the brain*. Toronto, Canada: Knopf.
Schmeck, R. R. (2013). *Learning strategies and learning styles*. New York, NY: Springer Science & Business Media.
Sevdalis, V., & Keller, P. E. (2011). Captured by motion: Dance, action understanding, and social cognition. *Brain and Cognition, 77*(2), 231–236. https://doi.org/10.1016/j.bandc.2011.08.005
Sievers, B., Polansky, L., Casey, M., & Wheatley, T. (2013). Music and movement share a dynamic structure that supports universal expressions of emotion. *Proceedings of the National Academy of Sciences, 110*(1), 70–75. https://doi.org/10.1073/pnas.1209023110
Smallwood, J., Brown, K., Baird, B., & Schooler, J. W. (2012). Cooperation between the default mode network and the frontal-parietal network in the production of an internal train of thought. *Brain Research, 1428*, 60–70. https://doi.org/10.1016/j.brainres.2011.03.072
Stein, M. B., Slavin-Mulford, J., Siefert, C. J., Sinclair, S. J., Smith, M., Chung, W., ... Blais M. A. (2015). External validity of SCORS-G ratings of Thematic Apperception Test narratives in a sample of outpatients and inpatients. *Rorschachiana, 36*(1), 58–81. https://doi.org/10.1027/1192-5604/a000057
Sternberg, R. J. & Zhang, L. (Eds.). (2001). *Perspectives on thinking, learning, and cognitive styles*. Mahwah, NJ: Routledge.
van den Daele, L. (1967). A music projective technique. *Journal of Projective Techniques & Personality Assessment, 31*(5), 47–57.
van den Daele, L. (2007a). *Music Apperception Test: Background, theory, and interpretation*. Las Vegas, NV: Psychodiagnostics. catalog.loc.gov Library Catalog: ML3838.V185 2007
van den Daele, L. (2007b). *Music Apperception Test manual*. Las Vegas, NV: Psychodiagnostics. catalog.loc.gov Library Catalog: ML3838.V185 2007
van den Daele, L. (2007c). *Music Apperception Test* [DVD]. Las Vegas, NV: catalog.loc.gov Library Catalog RZC 0159
van den Daele, L. (2014). The Music Apperception Test: Coding, research, and application. *Rorschachiana, 35*(2), 214–235. https://doi.org/10.1027/1192-5604/a000055
Webster, G. D., & Weir, C. G. (2005). Emotional responses to music: Interactive effects of mode, texture, and tempo. *Motivation and Emotion, 29*(1), 19–39. https://doi.org/10.1007/s11031-005-4414-0

Wehrwein, E. A., Lujan, H. L., & DiCarlo, S. E. (2007). Gender differences in learning style preferences among undergraduate physiology students. *Advances in Physiology Education, 31*(2), 153–157. https://doi.org/10.1152/advan.00060.2006

Westen, D., Blagov, P. S., Harenski, K., Kilts, C., & Hamann, S. (2006). Neural bases of motivated reasoning: An fMRI study of emotional constraints on partisan political judgment in the 2004 U.S. presidential election. *Journal of Cognitive Neuroscience, 18*(11), 1947–1958. https://doi.org/10.1162/jocn.2006.18.11.1947

Whissell, C. (2009). Using the revised dictionary of affect in language to quantify the emotional undertones of samples of natural language. *Psychological Reports, 105*(2), 509–521. https://doi.org/10.2466/PR0.105.2.509-521

Zvyagintsev, M., Clemens, B., Chechko, N., Mathiak, K. A., Sack, A. T., & Mathiak, K. (2013). Brain networks underlying mental imagery of auditory and visual information. *European Journal of Neuroscience, 37*(9), 1421–1434. https://doi.org/10.1111/ejn.12140

Received October 18, 2016
Revision received September 1, 2017
Accepted September 17, 2017
Published online May 9, 2018

Leland van den Daele
Professor Emeritus of Clinical Psychology
California Institute of Integral Studies
1453 Mission Street
San Francisco, CA 94103
USA
lvandendaele@ciis.edu

Summary

This project comprised two studies: first, the comparison of the relative performance of 26 professional dancers with 26 nondancers on the Music Apperception Test (MAT; van den Daele, 2014); second, the comparison of dancers' performance on the MAT Short Form with selected cards from the Thematic Apperception Test (TAT; Murray, 1943). The MAT Short Form asks respondents to "tell a story to the music" to compositions written to represent four basic emotions (love, guilt, excitement, and fear). Four TAT cards were selected that elicit similar emotions. Following standard TAT instructions (Murray, 1943), participants were asked, "What is happening in the picture? What happened before? How are people in the picture feeling? How are they thinking? How does everything turn out in the end?"

In the first study, dancers were significantly quicker and more fluent in storytelling than a comparison group matched for gender and age. On average, dancers were approximately three times quicker to respond than matched controls, while male dancers were approximately two and one-half times more fluent than male nondancers. Dancers were particularly responsive to the movement and mood conveyed by music tempo, rhythm, and voice that brought forth associated feeling, sensation, and imagery. Criterion-based evaluation of dancers' stories found narratives highly congruent with music mood. The professional practice of dance appeared to attune its practitioners to rapid assessment and fluent response to music meaning.

In the second study that compared dancers' MAT and TAT responses, fluency to the TAT was two times more variable than to the MAT. Approximately half the dancers were significantly more fluent on the MAT than the TAT, while the other half were significantly more fluent on the TAT than the MAT. The stories told to the MAT and TAT seemed to reflect different mental processes. MAT stories involved bodily movement, sensation, feeling, personal memory, and imagery akin to dream material while TAT stories were reflective and deliberative drawing from social and personal experience and scripts. In comparison with one another, the MAT elicited free fantasy, and the TAT engaged social cognition and explanation.

The results were interpreted as consistent with differences observed in neurological studies of auditory and visual processing, educational studies of modality preference, and the cognitive style literature. The MAT provided an assessment tool that appeared to complement the TAT in personality appraisal.

Résumé

Ce projet comprenait deux études: premièrement, la comparaison de la performance relative de 26 danseurs professionnels à 26 non-danseurs sur le Test d'Apperception de Musique (MAT, van den Daele, 2014); Deuxièmement, la comparaison de la performance des danseurs sur le MAT Short Form avec les cartes sélectionnées du Thematic Apperception Test (TAT; Murray, 1943). Le MAT Short Form demande aux répondants de «raconter une histoire à la musique» à des compositions écrites pour représenter quatre émotions de base (amour, culpabilité, excitation et peur). Quatre cartes TAT ont été sélectionnées qui suscitent des émotions similaires. Suivant les instructions TAT standard (Murray, 1943), on a demandé aux participants: « Qu'est-ce qui se passe sur l'image? Qu'est-il arrivé avant? Comment se sentent les gens dans l'image? Comment pensent-ils? Comment tout se déroule-t-il à la fin? »

Dans la première étude, les danseurs étaient significativement plus rapides et plus courant-ment parlants que le groupe de comparaison correspondant au genre et à l'âge. En moyenne, les danseurs étaient environ trois fois plus rapides à répondre que les témoins appariés, tandis que les danseurs masculins parlaient environ deux fois et demi plus couramment que les hommes qui ne faisaient pas de danse. Les danseurs étaient particulièrement sensibles au movement et à l'humeur transmis par le tempo, le rythme et la voix de la musique, ce qui a provoqué des sentiments, des sensations et des images associées. L'évaluation fondée sur le critère des histoires des danseurs a révélé des récits hautement congruents avec l'humeur musicale. La pratique pro-fessionnelle de la danse semblait accorder à ses praticiens une évaluation rapide et une réponse fluide à la signification de la musique.

Dans la deuxième étude qui a comparé les réponses MAT et TAT des danseurs, la fluidité vers le TAT était deux fois plus variable que pour le MAT. Environ la moitié des danseurs était beaucoup plus fluide sur le MAT que le TAT, tandis que l'autre moitié était beaucoup plus fluide sur le TAT que le MAT. Les histoires racontées au MAT et au TAT semblaient refléter différents processus mentaux. Les histoires MAT ont impliqué le mouvement corporel, la sensation, le sentiment, la mémoire personnelle et les images semblables au matériel de rêve, tandis que les histoires TAT étaient réfléchies et le tirage délibératif de l'expérience et des scripts sociaux et personnels. Le MAT a suscité une fantaisie libre, et le TAT a engagé une connaissance sociale et une explication.

Les résultats ont été interprétés comme compatibles avec les différences observées dans les études neurologiques du traitement auditif et visuel, les études pédagogiques sur la preference de la modalité et la littérature sur le style cognitif. Le MAT a fourni un outil d'évaluation qui a paru compléter le TAT dans l'évaluation de la personnalité.

Resumen

Este proyecto constaba de dos estudios: Primero, la comparación del desempeño relativo de 26 bailarines profesionales con 26 no bailarines en la Prueba de Apercepción Musical (MAT, van den Daele, 2014); En segundo lugar, la comparación del rendimiento de los bailarines en el MAT Short Form con las tarjetas seleccionadas de la Prueba de Apercepción Temática (TAT, Murray, 1943). El MAT Short Form pide a los encuestados que "cuenten una historia a la música" a composiciones escritas para representar cuatro emociones básicas (amor, culpa, emoción y miedo). Se seleccionaron cuatro tarjetas TAT que provocan emociones similares. Siguiendo las instrucciones estándar de TAT (Murray, 1943), se preguntó a los participantes: "¿Qué está sucediendo en la imagen? ¿Qué pasó antes? ¿Cómo se sienten las personas en la imagen? ¿Cómo están pensando? ¿Cómo acaba todo al final?"

En el primer estudio, los bailarines fueron significativamente más rápidos y más fluidos en la narración que un grupo de comparación emparejado por género y edad. En promedio, los bailarines eran aproximadamente tres veces más rápidos de responder que los controles emparejados, mientras que los bailarines eran aproximadamente dos veces y media más fluidos que los hombres no bailarines. Los bailarines eran particularmente sensibles al movimiento y al humor transmitidos por el tempo, el ritmo y la voz de la música que produjeron sensación, sensación e imágenes asociadas. La evaluación basada en criterios de las historias de los bailarines encontró narrativas altamente congruentes con el estado de ánimo de la música. La práctica profesional de la danza pareció sintonizar a sus practicantes con la evaluación rápida y la respuesta fluida al significado de la música.

En el segundo estudio que comparó las respuestas MAT y TAT de los bailarines, la fluidez al TAT fue dos veces más variable que al MAT. Aproximadamente la mitad de los bailarines eran significativamente más fluidos en el MAT que el TAT, mientras que la otra mitad era significativamente más fluida en el TAT que el MAT. Las historias contadas al MAT y al TAT parecían reflejar diferentes procesos mentales. MAT contó con movimientos corporales, sensación, sentimiento, memoria personal e imágenes similares al material de los sueños, mientras que las historias de TAT eran reflexivas y deliberativas, basadas en la experiencia y los guiones sociales y personales. En comparación entre sí, el MAT generó fantasía libre, y el TAT involucró la cognición social y la explicación.

Los resultados fueron interpretados como consistentes con las diferencias observadas en estudios neurológicos de procesamiento auditivo y visual, estudios educativos de preferencia de modalidad y la literatura de estilo cognitivo. El MAT proporcionó una herramienta de evaluación que parecía complementar el TAT en la evaluación de la personalidad.

要約

プロのダンサーの音楽統覚検査と主題統覚検査（TAT）の異なった遂行

　本研究課題は2つの研究から構成されている。第一の研究は、26名のプロのダンサーと26名のプロのダンサーではない人の音楽統覚検査（MAT; van den Daele, 2014）への反応の相対比較である。第二は、主題統覚検査（TAT; Murray, 1943）から選ばれた図版への反応を、MAT短縮版への反応と比較することである。MAT短縮版は反応者に"この音楽に対して物語をつくって"、4つの基本的な情緒（愛、罪悪感、興奮、恐れ）をあらわすように文章を書く、ように求める。類似した情緒を引き出すために4枚のTAT図版が選ばれた。標準的なTATの教示（Murray, 1943）の後、研究への参加者は"この絵の中では何が起こっていますか？この前には何がありましたか？絵の中にいる人はどのように感じていますか？彼らは何を考えていますか？結局、最終的にはどうなりますか？"を尋ねられた。

第一の研究では、ダンサーは年齢と性別を対応させた比較群よりも有意により早くよりなめらかに物語を話した。平均的にダンサーはおよそ対応している統制群に比較して3倍速かった、一方、男性のダンサーは男性のダンサーではない群に比較して2.5倍なめらかに物語を話した。ダンサーは特に、4つの関連する感情や感覚やイメージを伝える音楽のテンポやリズムや声によって伝達される運動やムードによく反応した。ダンサーの物語の基準にもとづいた評価によると、語りは音楽のムードに高度に一致していた。ダンスの職業的な実践は、音楽の意味を素早く査定し頻繁に反応するように実践家に同調させるようである。

ダンサーのMATとTATの反応を比較した第二の研究では、MATに比較してTATでは2倍以上の流暢さで反応していた。おおよそダンサーの半分がTATよりもMATで流暢に反応していたが、その一方でもう半分はMATよりもTATの方がより頻繁に反応していた。MATとTATに語られた物語は、異なった精神課程を反映しているように見えた。MATの物語は、身体の運動や感覚、感情、個人的な記憶、夢の素材と同じ心象を含んでおり、一方でTATの物語は、社会的あるいは個人的な経験やスクリプトの思慮深くて慎重な描写であった。TATと比較すると、MATは自由な空想を引き出し、TATは社会的認知と説明がなされていた。

本研究の結果は、聴覚情報処理と視覚情報処理の生理学的研究や、感覚モダリティの好みの教育における研究、認知スタイルの文献の中に見いだされる差異と一致していると解釈された。MATはパーソナリティの評価において、TATを補完するようなアセスメント・ツールとなっているようであった。

Original Article

The Italian Translation of Exner's FQ Tables

Need for a Critical Edition and for a Shared Standard

Luca Angelino and Alessandra Ciliberti

Rorschach Lab, Milan, Italy

Abstract: The article takes into consideration the four Italian translations (2003, 2007, 2016, 2017) of the Rorschach Comprehensive System Form Quality Tables (Exner, 2001), with reference to the original English version, highlighting the urgency to verify a number of possible errors that – if proven – would be necessary to rectify. In light of these considerations, we underline the need for an Italian critical edition, as a step toward a shared standard for a scientific instrument that must insure uniformity of results among Comprehensive System users.

Keywords: intercoder agreement, FQ tables, Rorschach, translation, validity

In Exner's Comprehensive System (CS), the Form Quality (FQ) tables represent a technical instrument essential in the coding process of Rorschach protocols. A code that expresses the *appropriateness* of the response – i.e., how much a response is to be considered *accurate* (*goodness of fit*) and/or *conventional* (*frequency*) – is attributed to each Rorschach answer, directly or by extrapolation, starting from the consultation of these tables.

The indices calculated with these codes (see *Mediation Cluster*) will ultimately allow the examiner to evaluate to which extent the subject is able to keep in contact with reality.

A delicate and relevant step for the assessment is in play: a refined evaluation regarding the subject's *reality testing* (Rapaport, Gill, & Schafer, 1946), and thus the "normal" versus "pathological" personality functioning (Rorschach, 1921; Weiner, 1966).

Over a time-frame of 30 years, the Rorschach Workshops have taken on the challenging task of constructing these tables. They were initially created on the basis of more than 26,000 responses from 1,200 protocols (Exner, 1974); today, in its fourth revision (Exner, 1986, 1993, 2001), the FQ table relies on a database of 205,701 responses from 9,500 protocols.

It is from this wide database that an essential list has been selected – to act as a reference unit – currently comprising 5,018 items, ordered by card and location, each one associated with an FQ code that can be *ordinary* (*FQo*, accurate *and* conventional), *unusual* (*FQu*, accurate but unconventional), or *minus* (*FQ-inaccurate*).[1]

The reference list currently used was published for the first time by J. E. Exner Jr. (2001).[2]

The Rorschach Research Council (RRC) – the advisory board created by Exner in 1997 with the goal of advancing the development of the CS, to promote research and to evaluate method upgrades – discussed, between 2001 and 2005, a list of 298 changes for a new edition of the FQ tables. However, Exner's death (February 20, 2006) led to the freezing of the CS, which thus remains stuck in its latest version (2001).[3]

The original reference tables, therefore, should not be considered as a work free of "irregularities, inconsistencies, obvious omissions, and redundancies" (Meyer et al., 2011, Italian trans., 2015, p. 445), which Exner himself wanted to correct.

However, these tables are currently the only reference point and the *standard* tool for the evaluation of the FQ according to the CS in research, in clinical and forensic practice, and in Rorschach training (Fontan et al., 2013, p. 59).

---

[1] In addition to these three codes, the CS provides two further unlisted possibilities: FQ+ (ordinary forms, improved by an "unusually detailed articulation"), FQ *none* or *no form* (a coding for FQ is not entered in case of formless responses).

[2] In 2002 the same tables were republished in a separate edition (Exner, 2002). The tables appeared once more in J. E. Exner Jr. *The Rorschach: A Comprehensive System, Vol. 1*, 4th ed., John Wiley & Sons (2003a). Finally, in 2003, the CS FQ Tables were included in the database of the latest software release of RIAP 5 (Rorschach Interpretation Assistance Program, Exner & Weiner, 2003).

[3] As we know, after this freezing, some authors from Exner's teams (G. J. Meyer, D. J. Viglione, J. L. Mihura, R. E. Erard, and P. Erdberg) developed a new approach to the Rorschach method – the Rorschach Performance Assessment System, R-PAS (2011) – which, based on the heritage of the Comprehensive System, aims to update the method as per the latest research. In this system an important review of the FQ tables was carried out, based on the 298 changes suggested by the RRC and on international research aimed at evaluating the Form Accuracy (FA) of the Rorschach responses (G. Meyer, personal communication, December 22, 2015). The Italian translation of these tables is available in the text published in 2015 by Raffaello Cortina, *Rorschach Performance Assessment System* (Chapter 6, pp. 197–272).

Review of the Existing Translations and Need for a Critical Edition

In Italy, there are four different translations of the American reference text. Two of these have been published in print format by Franco Angeli (Exner, 2003b) and Raffaello Cortina (Lis, Zennaro, Salcuni, Parolin, & Mazzeschi, 2007). Both volumes have been widely diffused and are still in use.

The third version is included in the CHESSSS database (Fontan et al., 2013), an open-source software, the result of an international project supervised by Anne Andronikof, Past President of the International Society of the Rorschach and 0Projective Methods (ISR) and of the European Rorschach Association (ERA), now Comprehensive System International Rorschach Association (CSIRA).

While the present paper was under review, a new Italian translation of the FQ tables was published in print format (June 22, 2017) by Raffaello Cortina (Abbate & Porcelli, 2017).

In the following analysis, the ensuing conventional codes for the four translations have been used:

FA03 Exner, J. E., *Rorschach: Compendio per il sistema comprensivo*, Franco Angeli, Milan, 2003. This is the full translation of the *Workbook* (2001), edited by the *Accademia Italiana Rorschach* (Anna Maniezzi, Bruno Zanchi, Filippo Aschieri), the Institute thanks to which Exner's CS was brought to Italy.

RC07 Lis, A., Zennaro, A., Salcuni, S., Parolin, L., & Mazzeschi, C., *Il Rorschach secondo il Sistema Comprensivo di Exner*, Raffaello Cortina Editore, Milan, 2007. The Italian translation of the FQ tables will be found in the Appendix of the volume, which presents a series of Italian contributions to the CS and, in particular, the results of research that has been carried on since 1998, in order to establish the Italian norms for the CS. This important research work is the Italian contribution to the wider international project for the *Composite Adult International Reference Values* (Meyer, Erdberg, & Shaffer, 2007).

CH13 Fontan, P., Andronikof, A., Nicodemo, D., Al Nyssani, L., Guilheri, J., Hansen, K. G., & Nakamura, N., *CHESSSS: A free software solution to score and compute the Rorschach Comprehensive System and Supplementary Scales. Rorschachiana*, 2013, 34(1), 56–82. The translation of the FQ tables for Italy – which appeared in the third release of the software (CHESSSS 1. 21) and later corrected (2015, CHESSSS 1.33; CHESSSS 1.35; 2016, CHESSSS 1.47) – has been edited by Daniela Nicodemo, Manuela De Blasi, and Rosanna D'Arrezzo.

RC17 Abbate, L., & Porcelli, P., *Rorschach Comprehensive System*, Raffaello Cortina Editore, Milan, 2017. In the preface (p. VIII), I. B. Weiner presents the volume "enriched by an accurate Italian translation of the Form Quality items."

Four translations for a single reference text: Which is most appropriate to use for professional practice?

It is a question worth asking. But there is a second even more important issue: Is it correct for a scientific tool to be available in four versions inconsistent from one another?

To answer the first question, the four translations were compared with each other, with reference to the original text. While doing so, we ran into a series of discrepancies and different kinds of errors, which are described in detail in the following pages. In this context we define *error*, and not mere *inaccuracy*, as anything that could lead the coder to a wrong FQ coding decision. These errors – if confirmed by an accurate verification by the scientific community – should be corrected urgently.

Here, we present the results of our systematic analysis of the first 623 items of the FQ tables (corresponding to Rorschach Card I).

For the sake of clarity, we have classified the errors into 10 typologies:

Type 1 Simple translation errors.
Type 2 Errors in the selection of the most appropriate meaning.
Type 3 Literal errors.
Type 4 Insertion of semantic ambiguities not found in the original text.
Type 5 Wrong transcription of the FQ code.
Type 6 Wrong transcription of the card orientation symbol.
Type 7 Omissions.
Type 8 Incomplete translations, omitting important features.
Type 9 Additions.
Type 10 Addition of important features not found in the original text.

In Table 1 we summarize the evaluation of the errors found for Card I, comparing the four Italian versions with Exner's original text.

In the sample of 623 items out of 5,018 that comprise the FQ tables, we counted 133 errors in RC07, 46 errors in FA03, and 19 errors in RC17.

In the case of CH13, we believe it to be possible and desirable that the errors – fewer than in the other translations (17 errors out of 623 items of Card I) – be corrected in the later releases of the software, according to the goal of constant improvement inspiring the project since its foundation, unreservedly also shared

Table 1. Errors found in the four Italian versions

Version	Type 1 errors	Type 2 errors	Type 3 errors	Type 4 errors	Type 5 errors	Type 6 errors	Type 7 errors	Type 8 errors	Type 9 errors	Type 10 errors	Total	%
FA03	11	3	1	7	1	1	11	4	7	0	46	7.38%
RC07	11	3	6	6	16	7	70	9	5	0	133	21.35%
CH13	4	4	1	5	0	0	2	1	0	0	17	2.73%
RC17	4	2	0	2	1	0	4	0	4	2	19	3.05%

by us. CH13 must be considered a work in progress. However, we think that the CHESSSS version is the one used less: In fact, many colleagues use paper editions in combination with other scoring software (RIAP, ROR-SCAN) or counting by hand.

To be fair, this review is incomplete. We know that some Italian institutes that provide Rorschach CS training programs have created other versions "for internal use only" (thus unpublished).[4] It was neither possible nor perhaps useful to find such versions, but their existence in the Italian scientific landscape gives rise to important considerations on the fragmentation of the Rorschach practice in Italy.

On the basis of this review, the most appropriate answer to the question raised is: Rather than choosing among the different versions currently in use, a critical edition is essential to verify the different sources of error, with reference to the original text.

A more detailed overview of the errors, classified in the 10 typologies, could contribute to highlight the need for and the urgency of this critical edition. The following review should also prevent the consideration of the translation of FQ tables as a simple work: It is, on the contrary, a technical high-profile task, which requires plenty of time and more accuracy than the precision needed by an average-level translation. Furthermore, this kind of analysis stresses the need to maintain a critical attitude among Rorschach practitioners.

Type 1. Simple Translation Errors

This error occurs when the Italian word chosen by the translator is not found – in the different dictionaries consulted (*Il Ragazzini 2016*, published by Zanichelli; *Grande dizionario inglese*, Picchi, F., published by Hoepli, 4th ed., 2014; *Oxford-Paravia*, 3rd ed., 2010; *Hazon*, 2008, published by Garzanti) – among the available translations of the original English term. These translation errors should be the starting point for a new version.

- Sometimes we notice that they are caused by false friends: Card I, W, *FQu*, *Coat of Arms* = It. *Stemma*, translated as *Cotta d'Armi* [i.e., Chainmail, Armor] (FA03, RC07).
- In other cases, the error is less clear: Card I, W, FQ-, *Smile* = It. *Sorriso*, translated as *Sospiro* [i.e., Sigh] (RC07).

---

[4] We are aware of two of these versions for internal use only: the first, edited by IRPSI (Istituto italiano Rorschach e Psicodiagnostica Integrata), the second, edited by A. M. Maniezzi (Accademia Italiana Rorschach), who also worked on the FA03 translation.

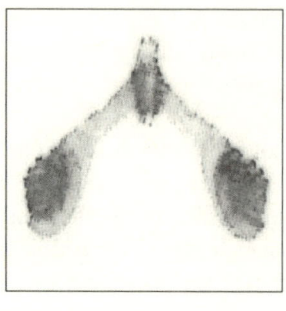
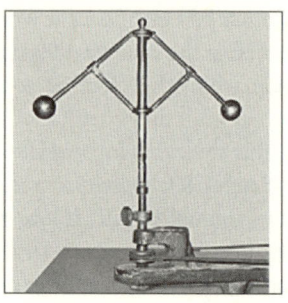

(1a) – Card X, D3   *(1b)* – Watt Regulator

Figure 1. Example from Card X (1a), (1b).

- Yet in other cases, we have to cope with technical details: Card X, D3, FQo, *Governor (on motor)*, translated by CH13 as *Generatore (motore)* – i.e., *Generator (motor)*. In similar circumstances the search engine Google Images could be helpful for the translator, as a visual dictionary.

In the specific case shown in Figure 1, assuming that the subject giving this type of response could be an engineer or a mechanic, we could translate: *Pendolo di Watt, Regolatore centrifugo* (i.e., *Watt's pendulum, Centrifugal governor*).

Type 2. Errors in the Selection of the Most Appropriate Meaning

These errors occur when the translator does not choose the most suitable term among different definitions consulted as possible translations of the same English word. This is perhaps the most insidious type of error and it is difficult to completely eliminate.

When the translation regards a work of fiction or an essay, the choice of the most appropriate meaning is usually suggested by the context of the sentence. In a list lacking context – as in the case of the Rorschach FQ table – the choice could be quite difficult.

Here, we propose four guidelines to cope with these cases.

First criterion: Some useful information can be taken from the perceptual context defined by the critical bits (Exner, 1996) of the relative location area. In short, we should ask which of the different meanings fits best with respect to the indicated location. This is a criterion that could be valid only in the case of items whose FQ are evaluated as *appropriate* (*FQo, FQu*). In fact, in the case of the *FQminus* – by definition – the critical bits are mostly ignored or infringed and

therefore the reference to the contours of the location area is useless or even misleading.
- Card X, D14, *Post*. Possible Italian meanings: *Posta, Corrispondenza, Posto (di lavoro), Accampamento, Palo, Messaggio* (i.e., *Mail, Correspondence, Job, Military camp, Pole, Forum message*). The D14 detail has a long and narrow shape: These characteristics represent the formal critical bits that would guide the interpretation of that portion of the inkblot. The fact that *Post* receives the *FQo* code means that the object is consistent with the critical bits: In other words, the item should be congruent, in the contours, to the location area. CH13 chooses *Posta* (i.e., *Mail, Letter*); we would choose *Palo* (i.e., *Pole*), on the basis of the perceptual context.
- Card I, Dd34 (orientation <), FQu, *Seal* = It. *Foca, Sigillo*. In the perceptual context: *Foca* (the sea animal) (RC07 and CH13). Translated as *Sigillo* (i.e., *Closure*) by FA03.

A *second criterion* could be the reference to the technical literature, in particular to the cases discussed in the classical texts (Exner, 2001, 2003; Exner & Erdberg, 2005; Weiner, 2003). If we find in an example or a protocol analyzed by one of these authors an item that coincides – for term used, location, orientation, and FQ code – with an unclear item, we could take the example itself as an indicative context.
- Card II, DS5, FQo, *Top*. Possible Italian meanings: Punta, Top (indumento), Trottola (i.e., Highest part, Upper part of a dress, Child's spinning toy). In the perceptual context (first criterion): It. Trottola (i.e., Spinning toy). However, since the shape of DS5 could also support the meaning Punta (i.e., Highest part), we have to turn to the literature of the sector. Exner (2003, p. 124) uses "Top," in the DS5 of Card II as the starting point for the extrapolation of the "Gyroscope" FQ code, commenting, "A gyroscope is a form of top." The second criterion is crucial here. Nevertheless, the term has been translated as Punta (CH13). FA03 and RC07 have been correctly translated as Trottola. Incidentally, we find the same error in the Italian translation of the FQ tables of the new R-PAS system (Meyer et al., 2011, Italian trans., 2015, p. 208, translation Cima, i.e., Pick).
- Card IV, D3, FQu, *Fan*. Possible Italian meanings: Ventilatore (i.e., Electric fan), Ventaglio (i.e., Hand fan). The perceptual context would lead to Ventaglio. In support of this choice, Exner and Erdberg (2005, p. 219) examine a protocol in which there is an Oriental Fan ("...the folds... is opened up," Case 9, Answer 6) corresponding to our puzzling item. Therefore, we choose

the meaning Ventaglio, while CH13 has Ventilatore (see also It. R-PAS Tables, p. 222).
- Card I, W, FQo, Moth = It. Tarma (i.e., Common clothes moth), Falena (i.e., Nocturnal butterfly). The item recurs 10 times in the FQ tables. In addition to the first two criteria (cf. Weiner, 2003, pp. 256–257) we could rely upon the clinical experience: Everything leads the translator to the option Falena. The word has been translated as Tarma (RC07).

A *third criterion* could be, as mentioned, the consultation of Google Images.

Basically, indexing the results by the search engine – working on a statistical basis – should provide mainly images referring to the most common perception, connected to the inspected word. However, this seems to be a weak criterion.[5]

For example, if we search in Google for the word *fan*, the images of electric fans appear on the first pages. This outcome does not lead us to change our mind about the translation referred to earlier.

In other cases, this criterion proved to be useful, but not conclusive.
- Card I, W (orientation ∨), FQu, Astrodome. Is it an astronomical dome (a sort of planetarium) or rather the Huston Stadium? Google Images guides us, with no doubt, to the second option, which is the choice of CH13. FA03 has Astrodomo, RC07 has Astronomo (i.e., Astronomer), the Italian translation of the R-PAS tables (Meyer et al., 2011, Italian trans., 2015, p. 198) has Planetario (i.e., Planetarium). However, if we only rely on this weak criterion, we are still in doubt.

Last but not least, a *fourth criterion* – only necessary in a limited number of uncertain and unsolvable cases – is the direct involvement of Rorschach experts in the translation, native American-English speakers. In our work for the critical edition, we have been supported by Mark J. Hilsenroth, PhD, Professor at the Adelphi University (NY), former member of the Rorschach Research Council (1997–2004). Thanks to his help, it was possible to select the right meaning in cases where no inner element could have definitively led to the decision.

---

[5] The weakness of this criterion is also due to intrinsic factors of the search engines functioning: in fact, the results partially depend on the date (the web is constantly changing), on the user's geographical location, on previous queries, and on other factors that personalize the output. Despite these limitations, which make the process weak from a scientific point of view, we have often used this further support as an accessory criterion. Since the Rorschach basically asks for a perceptual performance – relying on the visual channel – Google Images provides to the Rorschach practitioner a hint of what the visual perception more often connected with the searched word is, around the world.

Also, the doubt expressed earlier regarding Card I (W, Astrodome) has been solved – thanks to consultation with Dr. Hilsenroth – in favor of the Huston Stadium.

Taking into consideration the FA03 version, sometimes the translator seems to follow a criterion that we cannot approve: In the case of doubt, all the different meanings are included in the Italian list, without making a final decision. For example, FA03 has for Card I, W, FQo, *Moth*, both Tarma and Falena. The same principle leads to double *Hive (Insect)*, Card I, W, in *Alveare* (i.e., *Natural bees' nest*) + *Arnia* (i.e., *Man-made bees' nest*).

This criterion could be acceptable only in the case of tight synonyms, in order to make the consultation of the tables easier. In fact, for an Italian coder, it could be useful to find the lexical entry *Pelvi*, but also *Bacino*: This would facilitate the phase of extrapolation by similarity. However, in such cases, it would be recommended to use an internal cross-reference: *Pelvi* = q.v. *Bacino*, and, for this reason, to choose only one meaning with the correct FQ code. This is the only way to respect the original text, by keeping a one-to-one correspondence among the lexical entries, instead of multiplying them in the Italian translation.

Type 3. Literal Errors

This type of error occurs when the translator exchanges a word with another, which is phonetically or graphically similar, but totally different in meaning.

The cause of these errors is unknown. However, the outcome is quite different than typographical errors that are found in fiction texts or in newspaper articles, where the context of a sentence could easily suggest the most appropriate correction to the careful reader. In a list of items lacking context, it is virtually impossible to discover the error, unless we turn back to the English original source.

Moreover, these are serious errors, leading to a double misinterpretation: We could consider this error as an *omission* (Type 7 error: the correct item is missing) combined with an *addition* (Type 9 error: an item, missing in the original text, is added):

- Card I, DdS29, *FQo, Holes* = It. *Buchi*, translated as *Bruchi* (i.e., *Caterpillars*; RC07).
- Card I, Dd31, *FQ-, Hammer* = It. *Martello*, translated as *Mantello* (i.e., *Cloak*; RC07).
- Card I, Dd33 (orientation ∨), *FQu, Mushroom* = It. *Fungo*, translated as *Fuoco* (i.e., *Fire*; RC07).
- Card I Dd34, *FQ-, Face* = It. *Faccia*, translated as *Freccia* (i.e., *Arrow*; RC07).

- Card I, D2, *FQu*, *Leaf* = It. *Foglia*, translated as *Foglio* (i.e., *Sheet of paper*; FA03).
- Card III, D9, *FQu*, *Monster* = It. *Mostro*, translated as *Mosto* (i.e., *Must*, unfermented grape juice; RC07).

Type 4. Insertion of Semantic Ambiguities Not Found in the Original Text

A word with a univocal meaning in English when translated into Italian could give rise to confusion: The translator's duty should be to specify how the Italian word is to be understood.
- Card I, Dd22, *FQu*, *Labia* = It. *Labbra della vagina* (i.e., *Vaginal Lips*). The term *labia*, which cannot be confused with *lips*, has been translated as *Labbra* (FA03), without further specifications.
- Card I, D4, *FQu*, *Viola* = It. *Viola, strumento musicale* (i.e., the musical instrument; whereas in English the flower and the color are identified by the word *violet*); translated as *Viola* (FA03, RC07), without further specifications.
- Card I, W, *FQ-*, *Jellyfish* = It. *Medusa (animale;* i.e., the animal). Card I, W, *FQu*, *Medusa* = It. *Medusa (creatura mitologica;* i.e., the mythological creature). Both responses have been translated by CH13 as *Medusa*, without further specifications. In this case the lack of specification leads to a contradiction (same content, different FQ codes).
- Card X, D6 (orientation ∨), *FQo*, *Gorillas* = It. *Gorilla, due* (i.e., two). The specification seems to be necessary, because – in the Italian language – the word *Gorilla* is an invariable noun, a noun that does not change when inflected into the plural. The translation *Gorilla*, without further specifications (FA03, RC07, CH13), loses the evidence of the plural form.

On the contrary, when an ambiguous English word loses its ambiguity when translated into Italian, there would not be the need to translate the specification.
- Card I, W, FQ-, Pick (Guitar) = It. *Plettro* (in English we have to specify guitar, since the word pick also means a pointed tool, a toothpick, etc.). The word has been translated as *Plettro di Chitarra* (FA03, RC07, CH13), while *Plettro* would be enough.

However, it is evident here that the redundant information is simply useless and has no misleading implications on the coding process. We clearly have not counted such cases as errors.

Type 5. Wrong Transcription of the FQ Code

In some cases, we have noticed that an item in the Italian version has a FQ code that is different from the one found in the original text. More serious are those cases where an ordinary form (*FQo*) is wrongly downgraded to the level of a minus form (*FQ-*):
- Card I, W, *Face Fox* = *FQo*, transcribed as *FQ-* (RC07).
- Card I, W, *Crow* = *FQo*, transcribed as *FQu* (RC07).
- Card I, W, *Dragonfly* = *FQu*, transcribed as *FQ-* (RC07).
- Card II, D3 (orientation ∨), *Sun* = *FQo*, transcribed as *FQu* (CH13).
- Card V, D9, *Feet (Animal)* = *FQ-*, transcribed as *FQu* (FA03).
- Card X, D11, *Missile (with smoke or on pad)* = *FQo*, transcribed as *FQ-* (CH13).

Type 6. Wrong Transcription of the Card Orientation Symbol

In some cases, the Italian version does not provide the correct Card Orientation symbol.

The change in Card Orientation sometimes causes a dramatic variation in the perceptual gestalt of the inkblot. Therefore, in order to assign the tabulated FQ code to a response, the Card Orientation must also coincide with the indicated one:
- Card I, W (orientation ∨), *FQu, Tent, Circus Tent, Train (as D4 crossing a trestle), Spaceship*. RC07 omits the indication of the correct orientation for all the items.
- Card I, Dd34 (orientation <) *FQu, Ghost*. Both FA03 and RC07 omit the indication of the correct card orientation.
- Card VI, Dd21 (orientation ∨), *FQo, Head (Reptile)*. CH13 omits the indication of the correct card orientation.

Most likely, even in the original tables there might be similar errors. An evident example:
- Card VI, D1, FQo; Ship (reflected). In this case Exner himself omits reporting the correct card orientation (<), which could be inferred from a very similar response: Card VI, W (orientation <), FQo, Ship (reflected) with D3 as second object. In the R-PAS FQ tables (Cortina, 2015, p. 234) – for whose realization the authors have consulted the list of 298 modifications of the RRC – this error has been corrected.

A critical edition of the FQ tables should include, where possible, a warning or a solution to the errors detected in the original FQ tables.

Type 7. Omissions

Some items of the original list are missing in the translation. We do not refer here to the lexical entries that – strictly related to the Anglo-Saxon culture – would be hardly found in the Italian one: Astrodome; Plymouth Emblem; Doughnut; Chipmunk, etc. Removing these lexical entries could be correct, in view of an Italian standardization, but it would require ad hoc research. RC17 declares that some items have been eliminated from the Italian tables: among them "Plymouth Emblem [...] because too USA-specific" (see RC17, p. 349). We clearly have not counted this case as an error.

The most worrisome omissions regard those items with a relatively high frequency (above 2% in the American reference group), coded *FQo* (ordinary form). In fact, in the guidelines suggested by Exner (2003) for the extrapolation (FQ coding by extrapolation), the author specifies that, "in many instances, if a response does not appear in Table A [FQ Tables, ed.] it will probably be coded as unusual or minus" (Exner, 2003, p. 123). As a result, an item categorized as *FQo* in the original version, but absent in the Italian one, runs the risk of being coded *FQu* or even *FQ-*:

- Card I, W, *FQo*, *Human (winged or caped)* omitted by RC07. FA03 reports the item, but in an inexact version: *Umani, due, alati o incappucciati* (i.e., *Humans, two, winged or caped*).
- Card I, W, *FQo*, *Angels, 2 with D4 another object*, omitted by RC07.
- Card I, W, *FQo*, *Bug, Smashed*, omitted by RC07.
- Card I, W, *FQ-*, *Elves*, omitted by FA03.
- Card I, *FQo*, *People, 2, Dancing*, omitted by RC07.
- Card I, W, *FQu*, *Face, Skeleton (Animal)*, omitted by CH13.
- Card II, D2, *FQ-*, *Vase*, omitted by CH13.
- Card VII, DS7 (orientation ∨), *FQu*, *Head (Negative as in photo)*, omitted by RC07.

Note that omissions are one of the most common categories of errors, in particular for RC07 (for Card I, 70 errors out of 133 are omissions). RC07 sometimes omits entire blocks of responses: For example, the items related to Dd27 of Card II (5 items) and to Dd32 of Card V (12 items, out of which four are FQo) are totally missing.

Type 8. Incomplete Translations, Omitting Important Features

Here it is not the omission of an entire item, but some relevant elements in the description of the object. The incompleteness of the translation could compromise or mislead the correct comprehension of the item itself. On the contrary, when the incompleteness of the translation does not mislead the comprehension of the item, no error has been reported (i.e., omissions of irrelevant or marginal elements).
- Card I, Dd34 (orientation <), *FQu, Umbrella (Closed)* = It. *Ombrello (Chiuso)*. RC07 only has *Ombrello*. From a perceptual point of view, an open umbrella and a closed one are very different. We think that the lack of specifications leads one to automatically think of an open umbrella, the incorrect option.
- Card I, Dd24, *FQu, Human Figure (Lower half)* = It. *Figura Umana (Metà inferiore)*. RC07 only has *Umano (mezza figura;* i.e., *Human, Half)*. If there is no specification of which of the two halves we are referring to (upper or lower), it is more likely that we refer to the upper part: incorrect option.
- Card I, W, *FQu, Brain (Cross section)* = It. *Cervello (sezione trasversale)*. CH13 only has *Cervello, sezione*. The three types of anatomical sections (cross section; frontal or coronal section; sagittal section) create different perceptual gestalt.

Type 9. Additions

Sometimes we have found, in the Italian translation, some lexical entries that seem not to be included in the original text. This error is difficult to evaluate. In some cases, it could look like an error, but – in fact – it proves to be a result of the lexical entries multiplication that FA03 chooses, to face the problem of the variable meaning. When this happens, the apparent addition is nothing more than a double translation of the single original word. We have not reported any error for these repetitions. In other cases, on the contrary, no explanation could be found for the supernumerary lexical entries.
- Card I, W, *Islanda* (i.e., *Iceland*), *FQu*, absent in the original version, but added by FA03.
- Card I, D7, *Corona* (i.e., *Crown*), *FQo*, absent in the original version, but added by FA03.
- It is possible that *Islanda* depends on the alteration of *Island* (same location and FQ, It. *Isola*, while *Islanda* in English is *Iceland*) and Corona on the alteration of Crow (same location and FQ, It. *Corvo*, while *Corona* is *Crown*).

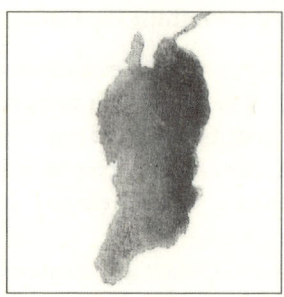 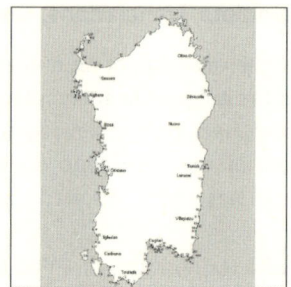

(2a) – Card X, D13 (CS)   *(2b) – Sardinia, Geographic map*

Figure 2. Example from Card X (2a), (2b).

- Card I, W, *Cervo* (i.e., *Deer*), *FQ-*, absent in the original version, but added by FA03 and RC07. We could suppose, in this case too, an alteration of *Door* (same location and FQ, It. *Porta*, while *Cervo* is *Deer*).
- Card VI, D3, *Vulva*, *FQ-*, absent in the original text, but added by RC07. We could suppose an alteration or a wrong translation of *Valve* (same location and FQ), item omitted by RC07.
- Card VII, Dd22, *Bandiera* (i.e., *Flag*), *FQu*, absent in the original one, but added by RC07.

As in the case of omissions, one could think of some licit additions. In a recent paper, Anna Maria Rosso wrote: "Perhaps the Rorschach scientific community needs more extensive Form Quality Tables, enriched with objects that are currently not included" (Rosso et al., 2015, p. 148). However, adding items to the CS FQ tables would require a specific research project on an Italian sample, comparable to the one carried out by the Scuola Romana Rorschach (SRR).

Just take into consideration the following classic case in Figure 2.

The response is not included in the American FQ tables. The SRR reports that the response *Sardegna* (i.e., *Sardinia*) to the D14, Card X (SRR System), occurs with a frequency of 2.02% for the Italian sample (Parisi, Pes, Cicioni, Amoros, & Collazo, 2003).

According to the CS criteria, this response should probably be coded *FQo*, but it is not possible to insert this lexical entry in the original list. In the case of an extrapolation through comparison between the two systems, one should declare with the utmost clarity the nature of the additions and the guiding criteria. This is anyway a methodologically questionable strategy due to the differences between the CS and SRR.

Type 10. Addition of Important Features Not Found in the Original Text

The last type of error – only found in the RC17 version – occurs when the translator arbitrarily adds some specifications that are not present in the original text.
- Card I, W (orientation ∨), *FQ-*, Pumpkin = It. *Zucca*. RC17 has *Zucca di Halloween* (i.e., *Halloween pumpkin*) but there is no trace of this specification in the American text.
- Card I, W (orientation ∨), *FQu*, Train (as D4 crossing a trestle): RC17 adds a note *(visto dall'alto;* i.e., *top view)*, which seems to be an arbitrary specification, since the original text has no indication about the point of view.

It is important to add some further considerations about the FQ tables integrated into the CHESSSS (2013) and the related Italian translation.

In our critical review work, we have extracted from the CHESSSS an Excel table in eight columns: identification number (a sequential number assigned by the authors), Card, Location, Orientation, original word, Italian translation, FQ code, content code. The last category does not regard the focus of this article. However, we noted a number of errors and inaccuracies in the CH13 content code assignation: Therefore, we have decided to include the column *contents* in the critical edition we are working on.

A second remark refers directly to the FQ review. Among the 10 typologies of errors listed earlier, the first four (and partially Type 8) are due to the translation work and could be corrected in the successive software releases by means of simple amendments.

However, the other typologies realistically depend on the original CHESSSS database, probably the starting point for all the other translations (in 10 languages to date). The correction, in this case, would require a verification of the English original version used as reference. Errors in this text have implications for all the other translations based on it and could be corrected only if we refer back to Exner (2001).
- For Card I, W, the original text (Exner, 2001) has *Face, Skeleton (Animal)*, *FQu*. In the CH13 English list this lexical entry is missing, therefore it went lost in all translations.
- At least in one case, an apparent error of translation proves to be created by a previous alteration of the English list. For Card I, D7, the original text (Exner, 2001) has *Bone, Osso, FQ-*. The Italian translation has *Rovina* (i.e., *Ruin*): a surprising incongruity. The puzzlement fades away when considering the CHESSSS English list, which has, instead of *Bone*, the literal error *Bane*, translatable as *Disgrazia, Sventura, Rovina, Veleno* (i.e., *Calamity, Misfortune, Ruin, Poison*). It is probable that all the translations have replicated this error.

In conclusion, taking into consideration all of these possible sources of error, the translator should pay particular attention during the realization of a new version.

At the Rorschach Lab, we have tried to create an Italian error-free version. This critical edition is under examination for a further check, to avoid possible errors that may have inopportunely passed the first checks.

The translation methodology we adopted in our work is the one known as *collaborative translation* or *collaborative check* (Douglas & Craig, 2007; Harkness, 2003; see also Chesher, 2014), modified to suit the specific material (a list of items lacking context). This work entailed the following steps:

1. Evaluation of the previous translations (FA03, RC07, CH13, RC17) with reference to the original English text and extrapolation of the possible errors in the 10 typologies illustrated earlier;
2. New integral translation by the first translator (draft file), with extrapolation of all the doubts (difficult cases);
3. Collaborative checking by the second translator: discussion of the difficult cases and their resolution, when possible, on the basis of the criteria specified earlier and, in particular, on the examples from the technical literature;
4. Extrapolation of the insolvable doubts, brought to the attention of a mother-tongue Rorschach expert;
5. Realization of a final draft (review file) with integration of the decisions on the difficult cases (adjudication), keeping trace of the decision process (documentation); and
6. Full check by the second translator.

The final result – although still to be refined – seems to be encouraging.

A further step obviously concerns the availability of this tool for all users of the Rorschach CS in Italy.[6]

Such a critical edition will always be open to further checks and reviews, in view of the utmost rigor and clinical functionality of the tool.

Our first idea was to offer this work to our students "for internal use only," but – while carrying on this work – we have changed our point of view.

We have reached now the heart of the second, still-pending, question: Is it correct for a scientific tool to exist in three/four/multiple versions that are inconsistent with one another?

---

[6] It is important to remember that the CS FQ tables are under copyright (Rorschach Workshops, Asheville, NC).

On the Way to an Italian Shared Standard

We have known for some time that our colleagues, using the Rorschach CS in their professional practice, are certainly aware of errors in the Italian reference translations. However, we feel that the real extent of these errors has often been ignored or underestimated, also because it is only verifiable through systematic research. To this point, we do not know about any other research undertaken in this direction.

In some cases, as mentioned, this awareness has led to local versions for personal use only, where a portion of the errors has probably been corrected.

Such a choice on the one hand guarantees a more reliable tool for the ones who use a "correct" version, while on the other hand it leads to an inadvisable fragmentation in the Rorschach practice.

In other words, the multiplication of the FQ table translations leads to a decrease in intercoder agreement with the addition of an amount of variance attributable only to divergences among translators. In fact, the four Italian translations only agree on 474 items out of 623 for Rorschach Card I (76.08%). It seems to be an unacceptable option for a scientific tool that should guarantee homogeneity and replicability of the results among Rorschach coders.

We think of our work as forensic psychological consultants often involved as auxiliaries in technical consultancies and expertise. Someone could legitimately ask if we can consider valid and reliable a Rorschach Structural Summary influenced by a decision regarding which translation to use, made by the examiner.

We can answer to this hypothetical interlocutor that an appropriate study would be necessary in order to evaluate the extent to which the errors affect the test's outcome.

In any case the principle underlying this objection is valid, because standardization of procedures and tools is essential in scientific work. Exner himself worked tirelessly for over 30 years to provide the Rorschach method with rigorous foundations.

Donald J. Viglione wrote in the introduction of his *Rorschach Coding Solutions* (2002, p. VII): "Good science and practice demand consistency and standards for administration and scoring."

It seems that the CHESSSS team also shares this concern when describing the specific approach to the FQ tables in the CHESSSS (op. cit. p. 59). Among the three aims stated in that context, two of them regard specifically the creation of a shared standard: "Create a reference system for FQ items; standardize the reference system for multiple languages."

The guiding attitude of our project is very similar. Moreover, we want to underline that, in order to reach this standard, two steps are required that could not be taken for granted:
1. The creation of a critical edition (in the acceptation used in philology and in textual criticism); and
2. The promotion of a widespread awareness among the final users of the tool, fostered by institutional statements in the suitable locations.

As we write this article, a careful evaluation of the stimulus material – the 10 Rorschach inkblots – is currently underway.

At present, different sets of Rorschach Test Plates are available on the market, giving rise to doubts about the possibility to use the reproductions alternative to the *historic standard*, which is provided by Verlag Hans Huber, now part of the Hogrefe group.

The International Society of the Rorschach and Projective Methods (ISR; Nakamura, 2014) has made this point very clear by publishing the *Guidelines for the Use of Rorschach® Test Plates,* where they state:

> The only Rorschach® Test plates authorized by the ISR for use in Rorschach diagnostics are produced exclusively by the Swiss publisher Hogrefe AG (formerly Verlag Hans Huber) [...] Unauthorized, imitation inkblot test plates sold by other publishers are not and cannot be considered reliable by the ISR and the scientific community.[7]

For those who use Exner's CS, we believe that a similar reasoning should be valid also for the second fundamental working instrument: the Rorschach CS FQ table. We hope that a national standard for the CS FQ tables – approved at institutional level, in this case the Comprehensive System International Rorschach Association (CSIRA/ARISI) – will be defined for each country.

In 2001, Piero Porcelli and Paola Appoggetti wrote (Exner, Porcelli, & Appoggetti, 2001, p. 15):

> The need to document the validity and the reliability of the Rorschach is not so much taken into consideration in the current clinical practice of the Italian psychologists, since few are the normative rules on the use of tests. For example, there are no official guidelines in this field from the reference institution, there is no requirement to give evidence of forensic admissibility

---

[7] Full text available on the ISR website at http://www.rorschach.com/the-rorschachr-test/guidelines.html

in the use of this or that test (Porcelli, 2001). On the contrary, the US system has a very different standard, requiring psychologists to comply with clear conditions.

Now, things are gradually changing. In the past few years, especially in the legal and forensic field, some authoritative guidelines have been created, also regarding the Rorschach (cfr. Centro Italiano Psicodiagnostica Integrata, 2014).

Following this line of thought, we have decided to work on a critical edition of the CS FQ tables for Italy. However, although such a work could be the result of the initiative of a single professional, the sharing of a standard follows different paths that we cannot, and we do not want to, walk alone.

Moreover, we hope that our effort put into the work of a faithful translation will not go lost but could indeed become a step in the direction for this standard in which we firmly believe.

Acknowledgments

We would like to express our gratitude to Mark J. Hilsenroth – PhD, Professor, Adelphi University (NY) – for all his valuable advice that has contributed to the solution of doubts in translation. A debt of gratitude is also owed to Luca Visconti – Open Gate s.r.l. CEO – for his IT support in our project.

References

Abbate, L., & Porcelli, P. (2017). *Rorschach Comprehensive System*. Milan, Italy: Raffaello Cortina Editore.
Chesher, T. (2014). *"Can we just check it?" Guidelines for checking of health/medical translations*. Gladesville, Australia: Multicultural Health Communication Service Retrieved from http://www.mhcs.health.nsw.gov.au/services/translation/pdf/GuidelinesForChecking.pdf
Centro Italiano Psicodiagnostica Integrata (2014). Linee guida per l'utilizzo della psicodiagnostica Rorschach in ambito forense [Guidelines for the use of Rorschach psychodiagnostics in court] In Linee guida per l'utilizzo della psicodiagnostica Rorschach in ambito forense. In R. Caporale & L. Roberti (Eds.), *Il test di Rorschach in ambito clinico e giuridico-peritale* (pp. 167–170). Milan, Italy: Franco Angeli.
Douglas, S. P., & Craig, C. (2007). Collaborative and iterative translation: An alternative approach to back translation. *Journal of International Marketing, 15*(1), 30–43.
Exner, J. E., Jr. (1974). *The Rorschach: A Comprehensive System. Vol. 1*. New York, NY: Wiley.
Exner, J. E., Jr. (1986). *The Rorschach: A Comprehensive System. Vol. 1: Basic foundations* (2nd ed.). New York, NY: Wiley.
Exner, J. E., Jr. (1993). *The Rorschach: A Comprehensive System. Vol. 1: Basic foundations* (3rd ed.). New York, NY: Wiley.

Exner, J. E., Jr. (1996). Critical bits *and the Rorschach response process*. *Journal of Personality Assessment, 67*(3), 464–477.
Exner, J. E., Jr. (2001). *A Rorschach workbook for the Comprehensive System* (5th ed.). Asheville, NC: Rorschach Workshops.
Exner, J. E., Jr. (2002). *Rorschach form quality pocket guide* (3rd ed.). Asheville, NC: Rorschach Workshops.
Exner, J. E., Jr. (2003a). *The Rorschach: A Comprehensive System. Vol. 1: Basic foundations and principles of interpretation* (4th ed.). New York, NY: Wiley.
Exner, J. E., Jr. (2003b). *Rorschach: Compendio per il sistema comprensivo*. Milan, Italy: Franco Angeli.
Exner, J. E., Jr., & Erdberg, P. (2005). *The Rorschach: A Comprehensive System. Vol. 2: Advanced interpretation* (3rd ed.). New York, NY: Wiley.
Exner, J. E., Jr., Porcelli, P., & Appoggetti, P. (2001). *Il test di Rorschach secondo il sistema di Exner* [The Rorschach test according to the Exner's system]. Trento, Italy: Erickson.
Exner, J. E., Jr., & Weiner, I. B. (2003). *RIAP 5 (Rorschach Interpretation Assistance Program)*. Lutz, FL: Psychological Assessment Resources.
Fontan, P., Andronikof, A., Nicodemo, D., Al Nyssani, L., Guilheri, J., Hansen, K. G., & Nakamura, N. (2013). CHESSSS: A free software solution to score and compute the Rorschach Comprehensive System and Supplementary Scales. *Rorschachiana, 34*(1), 56–82. https://doi.org/10.1027/1192-5604/a000040.
Harkness, J. A. (2003). Questionnaire translation. In A. Harkness, F. J. R. Van De Vijver, & P. P. Mohler (Eds.), *Cross-cultural survey methods* (pp. 35–56). New York, NY: John Wiley & Sons.
Hazon, M. (2008). *Grande dizionario Hazon di inglese 2009* [Great Hazon English dictionary 2009]. Milan, Italy: Garzanti.
Lis, A., Zennaro, A., Salcuni, S., Parolin, L., & Mazzeschi, C. (2007). *Il Rorschach secondo il Sistema Comprensivo di Exner* [The Rorschach according to the Exner's Comprehensive System]. Milan, Italy: Raffaello Cortina.
Meyer, G. J., Erdberg, P., & Shaffer, T. W. (2007). Toward international normative reference data for the Comprehensive System. *Journal of Personality Assessment, 89*(S1), S201–S216. https://doi.org/10.1080/00223890701629342
Meyer, G. J., Viglione, D. J., Mihura, J. L., Erard, R. E., & Erdberg, P. (2011). *Rorschach performance assessment system. Administration, coding, interpretation and technical manual*. Toledo, OH: Rorschach Performance Assessment System, LLC.
Meyer, G. J., Viglione, D. J., Mihura, J. L., Erard, R. E., & Erdberg, P. (2015). *Rorschach performance assessment system. Somministrazione, siglatura, interpretazione e manuale tecnico*. Milan, Italy: Raffaello Cortina.
Nakamura, N., Executive Board, International Society of the Rorschach & Projective Methods (ISR) (2014). *Guidelines for the use of Rorschach test plates*. Retrieved from http://www.rorschach.com/the-rorschachr-test/guidelines.html
Oxford-Paravia (2010). *Il dizionario inglese-italiano, italiano-inglese* [English-Italian, Italian-English dictionary] (3rd ed.). Turin, Italy: Paravia.
Parisi, S., Pes, P., Cicioni, R., Amoros, C., & Collazo, A. (2003). *Elenco delle Risposte Volgari, Semivolgari e di buona forma per frequenza statistica* [List of Popular, Semi-Popular and Good-Form responses, according to statistical frequency]. Rome, Italy: Istituto italiano di studio e ricerca psicodiagnostica Scuola Romana Rorschach.
Picchi, F. (2014). *Grande dizionario inglese* [Great English Dictionary] (4th ed.). Milan, Italy: Hoepli.
Ragazzini, G. (2016). *Il Ragazzini 2016*. Bologna, Italy: Zanichelli.

Rapaport, D., Gill, M., & Schafer, R. (1946). *Psychological diagnostic testing, Vol 2*. Chicago, IL: Yearbook Publishers.
Rorschach, H. (1921). *Psychodiagnostik*. Bern, Switzerland: Bircher.
Rosso, A. M., Camoirano, A., & Schiaffino, G. (2015). Are individuals in Rorschach nonpatient samples truly psychologically healthy?. *Rorschachiana, 36*(2), 112–155. https://doi.org/10.1027/1192-5604/a000052.
Viglione, D. J. (2002). *Rorschach coding solutions. A reference guide for the Comprehensive System*. San Diego, CA: Author.
Weiner, I. B. (1966). *Psychodiagnosis in schizophrenia*. New York, NY: Wiley.
Weiner, I. B. (2003). *Principles of Rorschach interpretation* (2nd ed.). Mahwah, NJ: L. Erlbaum Associates.

Recevied May 7, 2017
Revision received September 1, 2017
Accepted September 17, 2017
Published online May 9, 2018

Luca Angelino
Rorschach Lab
Milan
Italy
angelino.vigevano22@gmail.com

Summary

The present work was carried out with the aim of verifying the presence of translation errors in the four Italian versions of the Form Quality (FQ) tables for the Rorschach Comprehensive System and to evaluate their extent.

The results of the analysis carried out on the 623 items corresponding to Rorschach Card I highlight a variable proportion of errors in the four versions: 2.73% for the translation included in the CHESSSS software (2013, 2016); 7.38% for the version included in the Italian translation of *A Rorschach Workbook for the Comprehensive System* (Exner, 2001, Italian version, 2003); 21.35% for the translation included in the text *Il Rorschach secondo il Sistema Comprensivo di Exner, Manuale per l'utilizzo dello strumento* (Lis et al., 2007); 3.05% for the latest version, published in June 2017, in *Rorschach Comprehensive System* (Abbate & Porcelli, 2017). The errors found are of different kinds and have been classified into 10 typologies, to be as clear as possible: (1) simple translation errors; (2) errors in the selection of the most appropriate meaning; (3) literal errors; (4) insertion of semantic ambiguities not found in the original text; (5) wrong transcription of the FQ code; (6) wrong transcription of the card orientation symbol; (7) omissions; (8) incomplete translations, omitting important features; (9) additions; and (10) addition of important features not found in the original text.

The present study incidentally highlights the fact that similar translation errors are also present in the recent Italian version of the FQ tables for the Rorschach - Performance Assessment System (Meyer et al., 2011; Italian version, 2015).

The results of the study push the scientific community toward a thorough check of the quality of translation of a scientific tool representing a fundamental reference in clinical, forensic, and training settings. The Italian case calls on the international community to carry out similar checks on national translations.

A second concern arises from this survey. The existence of four translations inconsistent with each other of the only original reference text (FQ tables; Exner, 2001) in the Italian situation raises an even more radical methodological issue concerning validity and intercoder agreement. Since it was recently highlighted that it is necessary to determine on an international level which is the only authorized edition of the Rorschach Plates, we consider as fundamental the construction of a standard for the translation of the FQ tables, country by country, approved on an institutional level, so to ensure uniformity of results among Comprehensive System users. A similar goal should be included in the R-PAS users' agenda.

This work led the authors – through clarification of reasonable guidelines – to the construction of a critical edition of the FQ tables for Italy – not published yet – that will serve as a contribution to define such a shared standard.

Riassunto

Il presente lavoro è stato condotto allo scopo di verificare la presenza di alcuni errori di traduzione nelle quattro versioni italiane delle Form Quality Tables per il Rorschach Comprehensive System e di quantificarne la relativa portata.

I risultati dell'analisi effettuata sui 623 item relativi alla tavola I del Rorschach evidenziano una proporzione variabile di errori nelle quattro versioni: 2.73% per la traduzione inclusa nel software CHESSSS (2013, 2016); 7.38% per la versione inclusa nella traduzione italiana del *Compendio per il Sistema Comprensivo* (Exner, 2001, tr. it. 2003); 21.35% per la traduzione inclusa nel testo *Il Rorschach secondo il Sistema Comprensivo di Exner, Manuale per l'utilizzo dello strumento* (Lis et al., 2007); 3.05% per l'ultima versione pubblicata nel giugno 2017 in *Rorschach Comprehensive System* (Abbate & Porcelli, 2017). Gli errori riscontrati sono di varia natura e sono stati categorizzati, per maggiore chiarezza, in dieci tipologie: (1) errori di traduzione semplice; (2) errori nella scelta dell'accezione più appropriata al contesto; (3) refusi; (4) introduzione di ambiguità semantiche assenti nell'originale; (5) trascrizione errata della FQ; (6) trascrizione errata dell'orientamento della tavola; (7) omissioni; (8) traduzioni incomplete con omissione di elementi rilevanti; (9) aggiunte; (10) aggiunta di elementi rilevanti, assenti nell'originale.

Il presente studio evidenzia incidentalmente come simili errori di traduzione siano presenti anche nella recente versione italiana delle FQ Tables per il Rorschach – Performance Assessment System (Meyer et al., 2011; tr. it. 2015).

I risultati dello studio sollecitano la comunità scientifica ad una approfondita verifica della qualità della traduzione di uno strumento scientifico che costituisce un fondamentale riferimento in ambito clinico, formativo e forense. Il *caso italiano* invita la comunità internazionale ad effettuare simili verifiche sulle traduzioni nazionali.

Una seconda preoccupazione emerge da tale ricognizione. L'esistenza stessa, nel panorama italiano, di quattro traduzioni *fra loro incongruenti* dell'unico testo originale di riferimento (FQ Tables, Exner, 2001) solleva di per sé una questione metodologica ancora più radicale, relativa alla *validità* e all'*intercoder agreement*. Pertanto, come di recente è stata evidenziata la necessità di stabilire a livello internazionale quale sia l'unica *edizione autorizzata* delle tavole Rorschach, così riteniamo imprescindibile la costruzione di uno standard per la traduzione delle FQ Tables, nazione per nazione, riconosciuto a livello istituzionale, che garantisca uniformità di risultati agli utilizzatori del Comprehensive System. Un obiettivo simile dovrebbe rientrare nell'agenda degli utilizzatori R-PAS.

Il presente lavoro ha condotto gli Autori – mediante l'esplicitazione di ragionevoli *linee guida* – alla costruzione di una *edizione critica* delle Tavole per la Qualità Formale per l'Italia – ancora non pubblicata – che potrà costituire un contributo al progetto di definizione di tale *standard condiviso*.

Résumé

Cette recherche a été réalisée afin de vérifier la présence d'erreurs de traduction dans les quatre versions italiennes des Tables de Qualités Formelles du Rorschach en Système Intégré et d'en quantifier la portée.

Les résultats de l'analyse sur 623 qualités formelles de la planche I du Rorschach montrent un taux d'erreur variable dans les quatre versions: 2,73% pour la traduction incluse dans le logiciel CHESSSS (2013, 2016); 7,38% pour la version incluse dans la traduction italienne du *Compendio per il Sistema Comprensivo* (Exner, 2001, tr. it. 2003); 21,35% pour la traduction incluse dans le texte *Il Rorschach secondo il Sistema Comprensivo di Exner, Manuale per l'utilizzo dello strumento* (Lis et al., 2007); 3,05% pour la dernière version publiée en juin 2017 dans *Rorschach Comprehensive System* (Abbate, Porcelli, 2017). Les erreurs trouvées sont de natures différentes et ont été classées, pour une meilleure compréhension, en dix types: (1) erreurs de traduction simples; (2) erreurs dans le choix de la signification la plus appropriée; (3) fautes de frappe; (4) introduction d'ambiguïtés sémantiques absentes dans l'original; (5) transcription incorrecte de la qualité formelle (o, u, moins); (6) transcription incorrecte de l'orientation de la planche; (7) omissions; (8) traductions incomplètes avec omission d'éléments pertinents; (9) ajouts; (10) ajouts d'éléments significatifs et manquants à l'original.

La présente étude montre d'ailleurs que des erreurs de traduction similaires sont également présentes dans la version récente italienne des Tables de Qualités Formelles du Rorschach – Performance Assessment System (Meyer et al., 2011; tr. 2015).

Les résultats de l'étude engagent la communauté scientifique à procéder à un examen approfondi de la qualité de la traduction d'un outil scientifique qui est une référence fondamentale dans les domaines clinique, médico-légal et d'enseignements. Le 'cas italien' invite la communauté internationale à procéder à des vérifications similaires des traductions nationales.

Une deuxième préoccupation émerge de cette analyse. L'existence même, dans le paysage italien, de quatre traductions incompatibles avec le seul texte de référence original (FQ Tables, Exner, 2001) soulève une question méthodologique encore plus radicale concernant la validité et la fidélité inter-juges. Par conséquent, comme on a récemment souligné la nécessité de définir à l'échelle internationale une seule édition autorisée des planches de Rorschach, nous croyons qu'il est essentiel d'établir un standard pour la traduction des Tables de Qualités Formelles, pays par pays, reconnue au niveau institutionnel, qui assure des résultats cohérents pour les utilisateurs du Système Intégré. Un objectif similaire devrait figurer dans l'agenda des utilisateurs du R-PAS.

Le présent travail a conduit les auteurs - à travers la définition de lignes directrices raisonnables - à la construction d'une édition critique italienne des Tables de Qualités Formelles, encore inédite, qui peut contribuer au projet de définition d'un standard commun.

Resumen

Este estudio se llevó a cabo con el fin de comprobar la presencia de algunos errores de traducción en las cuatro versiones italianas de las Tablas de Calidad Formal para el Rorschach Sistema Comprehensivo y cuantificar su alcance.

Los resultados del análisis realizado sobre 623 item con respecto a la lámina I del Rorschach destacan una proporción variable de errores en las cuatro versiones: 2.73% para la traducción incluida en el software CHESSSS (2013, 2016); 7.38% para la versión incluida en la traducción italiana del *Compendio per il Sistema Comprensivo* (Exner, 2001, tr. it. 2003); 21.35% para la traducción incluida en el texto *Il Rorschach secondo il Sistema Comprensivo di Exner, Manuale per l'utilizzo dello strumento* (Lis et al., 2007); 3.05% para la última versión publicada en junio 2017 en *Rorschach Comprehensive System* (Abbate & Porcelli, 2017).

Los errores encontrados son de varias clases y se clasificaron, para mayor claridad, en diez tipos: (1) errores de traducción simple; (2) errores en la elección del significado más adecuado al contexto; (3) errores tipográficos; (4) introducción de ambigüedad semántica ausente en el original; (5) transcripción incorrecta de la Calidad Formal; (6) transcripción incorrecta de la orientación de la lámina; (7) omisiones; (8) traducciones incompletas con omisión de factores relevantes; (9) añadiduras; y (10) añadidura de factores relevantes, ausentes en el original.

El presente estudio destaca por cierto como errores parecidos de traducción están también en la reciente versión italiana de las Tablas de Calidad Formal para el Rorschach - Performance Assessment System (Meyer et al., 2011; traducción it. 2015).

Los resultados del estudio solicitan la comunidad científica a una comprobación exhaustiva de la calidad de la traducción de un instrumento científico que constituye una referencia fundamental en ámbito clínico, de formación y forense. El *caso italiano* pide a la comunidad internacional que lleve a cabo controles parecidos en las traducciones de cada país.

Una segunda preocupación surge de esta encuesta. La misma existencia, en el panorama italiano, de cuatro traducciones entre ellos incoherentes del único texto original de referencia (FQ Tables, Exner, 2001) plantea una cuestión metodológica aún más radical, con respecto a la *validez* y a la *fiabilidad inter-evaluadores*.

Por lo tanto, como se destacó recientemente la necesidad de determinar a nivel internacional cuál es la única edición autorizada de las láminas del Rorschach, así consideramos imprescindible la creación de una norma para la traducción de las Tablas de Calidad Formal, nación por nación, reconocida por las instituciones, asegurando resultados uniformes a los usuarios del Comprehensive System. Un objetivo parecido tendría que ser incluido en la agenda de los usuarios R-PAS.

Este estudio llevó los Autores – a través de la clarificación de *normas* razonables – a la construcción de una *edición crítica* de las Tablas por la Calidad Formal para Italia - no publicada todavía – que servirá como un aporte al proyecto de definición de dicha *norma compartida*.

要約

エクスナーの形態水準表のイタリアへの翻訳：校訂版と共有される標準の必要性

本研究はロールシャッハ包括システムの形態水準（FQ）表の4つのイタリア語版の翻訳の誤りの存在を確かめ、その程度を評価することを目的として遂行された。

ロールシャッハ第一図版に対する623の項目に対しておこなわれた分析は、4つの版の誤りの割合を明らかにした。CHESSSSのソフトウエアによる翻訳には2.73%であり、ロールシャッハ包括システムワークブック（Exner, 2001、イタリア版は2003）のイタリア語翻訳版には7.38%、Il Rorschach secondo il Sistema Comprensivo di Exner, Manuale per l'utilizzo dello strumentoのテキスト（Lisら, 2007）の翻訳には21.35%、2017年6月に刊行された、包括システムの最新版（Abbate & Porcelli, 2017）では3.05%であった。発見された誤りは多様であり、10の類型に分類された。それらは以下のようなものである。(1)単純な翻訳の誤り、(2)最も適切な翻訳の選択の際の誤り、(3)誤字、(4)原著の文脈には存在しない、意味の曖昧さの挿入、(5)FQコードの転載ミス、(6)カード方向の印の転載ミス、(7)省略、(8)不完全な翻訳、重要な特徴の省略、(9)付け足し、(10)原著の文脈にはない重要な特徴の付け足し。

本研究は、ついでながら、ロールシャッハ法の最新のイタリア語版のR-PASシステム（Meyerら2011、イタリア語版は2015）においても同様の翻訳の誤りがあるという事実を目立たせた。

本研究の結果は科学団体に、臨床や犯罪、訓練の現場において基本的な基準となるものを代表しているこの科学的なツールの翻訳の質を徹底的にチェックさせるように仕向けさせた。イタリア人の症例が国際的な団体に収集され、国家的な翻訳に同様のチェックを遂行させた。

この調査から2つ目の関心が生じてきた。イタリアの状況においては、たった一つのオリジナルの文献テキスト（エクスナー、2001の形態水準表）に一貫しない4つの翻訳が存在することで、妥当性とコード者間の一致に関するより根本的な方法論における問題を提起している。正当版と認められたロールシャッハ図版

が唯一であるという国際レベルの決定が必要であるということが注目されたのは最近のことであるが、形態水準表の標準版の構築が最も基本的なこととわれわれは考える。それは国際的に、協会のレベルで承認され、それによって包括システムの利用者において、結果の均一化を保証する。同様の目標がR－PAS利用者の課題にも含まれるべきであろう。

本研究は、合理的なガイドラインの明確化を通して、著者らに、これはまだ公刊されていないのであるが、イタリアの形態水準表の決定版の構築を導くことになる。そしてそれは、共有される標準を定義するものとしての貢献するであろう。

Original Article

SCZI or PTI – Schizophrenia or Psychosis?

A Follow-Up Study

Vera Campo[†]

Sociedad Catalana del Rorschach y Métodos Proyectivos (SCRIMP), Barcelona, Spain

Abstract: This paper attempts to illustrate the usefulness of therapy follow-up studies with the Rorschach, based on a particularly striking and difficult protocol (including Structural Summary 1 and 2), in which the two indexes pointed to either schizophrenia (Schizophrenia Index, SCZI) or a psychotic episode (Perceptual-Thinking Index, PTI) in an adolescent whose later development was distinctly positive. Implications of the interpretive process are discussed, of the use of both indexes in favor of the PTI, as well as of the danger of depending on single indexes or of using the Rorschach for psychiatric diagnosis.

Keywords: Rorschach, PTI, SCZI, psychosis, schizophrenia

The interest of this case resides in the possibility of observing a psychotic break with the Rorschach (and secondarily with the Wechsler) and to follow the subject's development – astonishingly positive – after 10 years of psychoanalysis, despite the positive Schizophrenia Index (SCZI) and Perceptual-Thinking Index (PTI) in the first and second Rorschach after 2 years of treatment.

The assessment was requested because this rather shy adolescent, good student and sportsman, beat up his family in a fit of fury. Electroencephalography (EEG) indicated a temporal dysrhythmia during hyperventilation, which disappeared later with medication. The psychoanalyst did not think that Alex had schizophrenia but rather that he had severe schizoid personality disorder.

SCZI or PTI?

On the basis of one of the most intriguing Rorschach protocols I have ever encountered and the subsequent positive development of the patient, in this paper I aim to illustrate some difficulties inherent in the use of Exner's (1990) "old" SCZI in comparison with the new PTI (Exner, 1997–2003; see Table 1).

Apart from this more technical aspect, I wish to emphasize the great usefulness of the Rorschach for understanding personality, well beyond its merely

Table 1. PTI and SCZI variables

PTI	SCZI
1. $XA+\%^a$ < .70 and $WDA\%^b$ < .75	1. $X+\%$ < .61 and $S-\%$ < .41 or $X+\%$ < .41 or $X+$ < .50
2. $X-\%$ > .29	2. $X-\%$ > .29
3. LVL2 Sp.Sc. > 2 and FAB2 > 0	3. Either $FQ-$> = FQu o $FQ->FQo + FQ+$
4. If R < 17 and $WSUM6$ > 12^c or R > 16 and $WSUM6$ > 17^d	4. $SumLv2$ Sp. Sc > 1 and $FAB2$ > 0
5. $M-$ > 1 or $X-\%$ > .40	5. Either $RAWSUM6$ Sp. Sc. > 6 or $WSUM6$ Sp. Sc. > 17
	6. Either $M-$ > 1 or $X-\%$ > .40

Note. PTI = Perceptual-Thinking Index. SCZI = Schizophrenia Index. [a]XA (Extended Form Appreciation% = All responses with $FQ+$, FQo, or FQu divided by R). [b]WDA (W, D Appropriate% = All W, WS, D, and DS responses with $FQ+$, FQo, or FQu divided by the sum of all W, WS, D, or DS responses). [c]If R < 17: for ages 5–7, $WSUM6$ > 16; for ages 8–10, $WSUM6$ > 15; for ages 11–13, $WSUM6$ > 14. [d]If R > 16: for ages 5–7, $WSUM6$ > 20; for ages 8–10, $WSUM6$ > 19; for ages 11–13, $WSUM6$ > 18.

normative, statistical, or diagnostic features, in a psychiatric sense. In other words, what is this personality's inner world like, how does this influence its functioning, and furthermore – if needed – how can this personality be helped? Also, in addition, this case attempts to illustrate the usefulness and richness of follow-up studies, for the Rorschach practitioner as well as for the patient and the therapist.

Since adopting the Comprehensive System (CS) in 1978 and having lived through several modifications of the SCZI, I was too often bothered by the many false positives identified with this index (see, e.g., Campo & Vilar, 1990, or Campo, 1993). Also, in my opinion, the PTI is simply more elegant in its construction.

To my mind the misidentification depends not only on the first two components of the SCZI ($X+\%$ < .61 and $S-\%$ < .41 or $X+\%$ < .50; $X-\%$ > .29), but also on the last one ($M-$ > 1). Despite coinciding with the view that impaired reality perception is pathognomonic of schizophrenia, and therefore also with the fantasy distortion represented by the $M-$ responses, these phenomena appear to be rather common among nonschizophrenic Argentine and Catalan subjects (Campo & Vilar, 2007), so that these aspects seem to merit further attention and discussion.

Experience with the second attempt of establishing norms for voluntary subjects in Barcelona and its surroundings (N = 517, 1999–2007), showed that the means for $X+\%$, $X-\%$, and $M-$ are quite different from Exner's and Erdberg's (2005–2007) norms for nonpatients (N = 450; see Table 2).

So different, that a rather obvious conclusion is suggested: If the SCZI is applied to this type of Catalan population (voluntary functioning subjects taken, so to say, off the street by students of the Barcelona Rorschach School), the rate of false positives will probably be high, since one of its characteristics is an apparently

Table 2. Comparison of Exner's and Campo & Vilar's data

Exner	Campo & Vilar
X+% 0.68, SD 0.11	X+% 0.54, SD 0.14
X−% 0.11, SD 0.07	X−% 0.21, SD 0.10
M− 0.23, SD [0.57]	M− 0.78, SD 1.08

much lower correct perception of reality – or just different from CS norms? – but which coincides with the majority of other international normative studies, including the M responses. In other words, the cut-off points for X+%, X−%, and M− responses might be, respectively, lower and higher if this aspect is to correctly identify the schizophrenic patient's failure to perceive reality correctly, at least in an average Catalan population. As to *Sum6* and *WSum6*, without considering Level 1 and Level 2 thought disturbances, it is true that the Barcelona voluntary sample scores higher on these two aspects than the CS nonpatient normative group. However, so do the Japanese and Belgian nonpatient samples. Therefore, even in this aspect of the former SCZI, false positives may slip through.

But I do wish to refer to one other important issue, the coding of the *M*− responses, in particular due to its diagnostic weight, emphasized both by Exner and by Smith, Baity, Knowles, and Hilsenroth (2001). The new PTI, in which *M*− continues to be > 1, does not solve the issue. Whenever an *M*− is coded, the perceptually negative aspect of the response depends on two alternative possibilities: (a) the movement is "impossible to see" because the form of the human shape is distorted; and (b) a part of the response, but not the human figure in itself, is "impossible to see" (as, e.g., on Card III, D1, where this is quite frequent: "Two women – D9 – fighting over a baby – D7 – like in the story of King Solomon," or "Two men – D9 – playing a double piano – D7 – concerto," etc.). In other words, the human form and movement are correctly perceived but another part of the response is not, thus spoiling the response's form level in the CS. This is quite a different matter as compared with responses in which the human figure and movement are in themselves distorted. It must be admitted that this not so unusual occurrence is difficult to differentiate with the current CS coding rules. Its interpretation, as usual, depends on the clinician's acumen and experience (see Campo, 2015).

Exner presents and interprets the PTI (Exner, 1997–2003, pp. 524–525) and at the end cites Smith et al. (2001) pointing out that they:

> Studied the efficiency of the PTI with a sample of inpatient children and adolescents. They calculated thought disorder indices from a behavior rating

scale and a self-report measure. They found that the PTI used categorically, was able to differentiate patients with and without elevated thought disorders on the other measures. (p. 525)

And they recommend the use of the PTI rather than the SCZI with younger subjects since the former "seems to be more related to behavioral ratings and self-report of thought disturbance than the SCZI" (p. 460).

To return to the beginning of this introduction to these two indexes, my objective is not only to share a striking Rorschach protocol and its author's development, but also to illustrate again the Rorschach's potency as an instrument that helps us to understand people with their assets and difficulties.

I also wish to point out that in the easily available references – *Journal of Personality Assessment* and *Rorschachiana* – in the last 10 years I did not find any articles dealing with these two indexes. With two exceptions: the Finnish paper (Kalla et al., 2002) and one of my own that I had forgotten (Campo, 2000), both in *Rorschachiana*. In the former, curiously and astonishingly, the SCZI was not very efficient in identifying schizophrenia, while in the latter the SCZI misidentifies too many not-psychotic or schizophrenic subjects. Once again, such results give support both to the change of name, that is, to the PTI, and to the well-known and important argument that the Rorschach indexes as well as the test itself are not to be used for psychiatric diagnosis.

Brief Report on 15-Year-Old Alex's History and the Reason for Consultation

Three months before consultation, Alex has taken an LP record from his younger brother, who demanded it back but Alex would not return it. The next morning the brother insisted and Alex then threatened to kill him and proceeded to beat him up brutally; when the father intervened, Alex knocked him down too and also beat his mother. The father then said he was calling the police and Alex stopped and went to sleep for the whole afternoon. During the following weeks he seemed obsessed and wrote terrible notes, but, full of suspicion, would not visit a psychiatrist; he did accept to have an EEG, a personality assessment, and to initiate therapy if this proved necessary at school's end.

About 1 year earlier he had experienced a period of black moods and punched his father when the latter reproached him. Sometime before the manifestations that led to consultation with his future psychoanalyst, and to the psychological assessment, Alex felt he was fat, dieted, and lost 10 pounds in 1 month. Unfortunately, this diet – prescribed by the family's general practitioner – contained amphetamine. Later, he went back to eating regularly.

As a small child (1 year old) when Alex cried he turned blue around the mouth, and also later when he became angry, but not often; usually he contained his rage until he exploded. Otherwise he was a sweet and quiet boy. He has a brother who is 3 years older than him, and one who is 3 years younger, of whom he is extremely jealous. Alex's development was normal. He had scarlet fever at the age of 4 years and rheumatic fever at age 12.

Alex is a very good student, exceedingly responsible, and always had the best grades. He has a profound sense of justice, does not compromise, tends to punish himself, and sometimes provokes his father in this sense (the father is violent too but usually controlled). He plays rugby and other sports, always violently.

Alex is not very communicative, is not interested in girls or parties, is more interested in ideas than in their expression, and his vocabulary is poor.

Assessment

Alex is a very good-looking, attractive, quiet boy. His attitude during the testing was distant but he collaborated seriously and well. During the Rorschach administration (see Appendix A) he seemed rather strange, but it was on the Object Relations Test (ORT; Phillipson, 1995) that I really began to feel scared because he sounded so peculiar, as if he were speaking from a distant, largely disconnected dream world, full of abstract ideas at times difficult to understand (see protocol in Appendix A).

Rorschach Interpretation

The structural data emphasize the great likelihood of schizophrenia (SCZI = 6) or another active psychotic state (PTI = 5), as well as of a major affective disorder (DEPI = 7). Although the logical sequence of interpretation reasonably points to starting with the cognitive triad, my impression is that affects together with object relations play the most significant role in Alex's protocol. Why? Because of sequence analysis. Therefore, some brief ideas regarding this essential and important part of the Rorschach interpretation will be presented first.

Alex "signs in" with a female symbol (I: R1, butterfly) and relates it to death, old violence (R2), and annihilation (R3), followed by confusion and flight (R4 = CONTAM).

Bloody, destructive, primitive affect, contradictory, confused feelings, and orality (Card II: R5, 6, 7), again followed by destruction (R8, 9), finally become organized into a much more structured but aggressive and severely split response (R10).

On Card III the unexpressed (retained C') "antique" hate emerges, only slightly disguised by socialized, formal, interpersonal relations (R11, P). The four responses to the next Card (IV) clearly show the dead aspects of the masculine image suggested by this card, and enhance his extreme pessimism (MOR = 13) and feelings of being damaged. The following four responses (V) point to sexual role confusion (R17) and violent splitting (R18, 19) – actually Bleuler's *Spaltung* – once more disguised by the first popular response (R16).

The sadomasochistic element is evident on Card VI (R20) with ensuing ruin and confusion (R21, 22, 23), surely pointing to serious problems in close contacts (no T, positive HVI) and, therefore, perhaps in the sexual sphere.

Card VII emphasizes the barrenness and loneliness (R25) – already mentioned in Card IV, R13 – and confusion (male instead of female faces and $F-$, R24) in his relation to the female image suggested by this card.

Although the impulse for achievement persists (VIII: active FM, R26), a positive aspect, Alex quickly becomes confused (R27) and morbid (R28) again. The primitive, disorganized, and destructive oral content is shown in one of his worst responses (IX: R29). Finally, on Card X some attempts at manic denial seem to emerge (R30), together with the innocence of R32, and he "signs out" with a hope of "renewal"? (R34, last response).

These rapid notes appear to coincide rather closely with the structural data to be enumerated, and add some flesh to that skeleton.

The fact that Alex habitually merges feeling with thinking (rigidly extratensive EB) and that his emotions are so unmodulated (6 Pure C, FC:CF + C = 3:12) makes his fit of rage easier to understand. It also explains his very exaggerated acceptance of less precise logic systems: his much too disturbed thinking (Special Scores), very low contact with and sense of reality (very poor *XA* and *WDA%*, and high $X-\%$), unconventionality (low P), and often quite primitive conceptualization (DQv = 10), aspects that suggest behaviors that disregard social demands and expectations. This is, moreover, complicated by the abuse of fantasy ($Mp > Ma$) and points to the possibility of delusional thinking, an aspect that seems evident on simply reading the protocol.

That situational stress (3m + 2Y) and terrible persecutory anxiety (Campo, 1979) and guilt ($m+C'+V+MOR$+Contents) limit his capacity for concentration and deliberate thinking is quite clear too. (In fact, a second assessment of intelligence [WAIS] 3 years later – after 2 years of treatment – shows a higher and more even level; see later sections.)

The fact that intellectualization – besides massive splitting, projection, devaluation, and projective identification (Cooper, Perry, & Arnow, 1988) – is still functioning, might be fortunate in this case, since it suggests the persistence of obsessive (more neurotic) defenses, although this mechanism is obviously failing and does not help Alex to deal realistically with his too intense emotional experiences.

Another negative prognostic aspect is his unusually good capacity for control (AdjD = +1), pointing to a pervasive stabilization of character traits; treatment will surely be long! But again, a positive implication exists too in his very rich and complex resources (EA = 22.5), even if the dilation of the EB may also signal a psychotic expansion, particularly on the flooded (6 pure C′, 3 pure C′[1]) affective side, but also in the realm of thinking (Special Scores).

Positive too, in this frightening protocol, is the marked avoidance of emotional stimuli (very low Afr) that seems to represent some awareness of emotional control problems – which he certainly has – and that at the same time point to Alex's (schizoid) not very communicative behavior (mentioned in the historical data). But at the same time Alex "swallows" (C′ = 11) a large part of the feelings he would like to express, which reinforces his emotional withdrawal, and also the potential for explosive reactions (also mentioned in the historical data).

It is clear that he is currently very distressed and suffering, much too involved in his experiences (low Lambda with too high blends), with intensely negative, painful, and confusing emotions and terribly pessimistic thoughts (MOR = 15), as well as having very low self-esteem, together with a truly serious depression (DEPI = 7). The "excessive introspection" (two vistas, one pure) may not be so excessive in this context, since without the guilt feelings mentioned before, he might be an inaccessible, perhaps psychopathic, very negativistic, oppositional, angry ($S = 5$) and crazy sort of "monster."

Alex's anger and hate, which make him feel alienated because he does not accept himself and which in turn determine the feeling of not being accepted, are evident in the fit of rage that led to the consultation, and certainly co-determine his difficulty in sustaining deep and close ($T = 0$) relations with others, especially the opposite sex (see follow-up data), as well as illustrating his intolerance and lack of compromise (mentioned in the history). Here the paranoid, hypervigilant style (HVI) appears to reinforce the negativistic and avoidant behavior and his extreme pessimism too.

Since Alex's self-image is largely based on imaginary rather than on real experience, also highlighting immature aspects of the self-concept and very distorted notions about himself and others, it is not surprising that he is greatly confused and concerned about his body (6 An+Xy, 5 with negative form

---

[1] The four instances of C.C′ combinations suggest panic reactions as well as the clash between the excessive internalization of feelings with their violent acting out. Also, this combination was found to be positively related to severe depression (Campo, 2003–2004).

level), a concern that may reflect hidden, destructive, and guilty sexual thoughts. (I did not learn about his foot fetishism until several years later; see follow-up data.)

Interpersonally, despite his suspicions, distance, and aggressiveness[2], the fact that he remains very interested in people, apart from the paranoid and controlling connotation, may be understood more favorably as a sign that objects continue to exist in his alarmingly destroyed and destructive inner world. Nevertheless, his oral dependence ($Fd = 2$) may also indicate his need to rely on others from whom he wishes to obtain sustenance but without coming into close contact.

Treatment is urgently necessary and will not be at all easy. The overall prognosis seems rather negative since diagnostically the SCZI and the PTI together with the feelings transmitted by the protocol do not appear to leave much room for hope of a complete recovery.

On applying the new Maladjustment Index (MI), this same impression holds, since Alex is positive on six of the seven items except for $AdjD < 0$.

Nevertheless, regarding Alex's analyzability, it should be pointed out that: (a) he is motivated for treatment because he is suffering ($D < AdjD$); (b) he is cognitively flexible (a:p); (c) he is very motivated to find solutions to problems (high Zf and W) even though his aspirations seem to be exceedingly high (W:M); (d) he is interested in other people; (e) he has access to affects even if he represses his feelings (C') and withdraws (low Afr); (f) he is very intelligent ($DQ+$ vs. DQo), more than the first WAIS indicated (see Table 3); and (g) he has rich and complex resources. The repetition of the Rorschach would be very useful.

As regards treatment planning, since it was going to be psychoanalysis, treatment would evidently be prolonged and justifiably so in view of Alex's current state. It is well known that this type of treatment can diminish anxiety and depression, emotional withdrawal, and a too explosive affectivity, also taking the help of medication into consideration. With dynamic therapy reality contact and self-esteem improve, and intellectualization and thought disturbances diminish. The analyst would initially have to pay more attention to subjective distress than to his pessimistic thinking.

The Bender-Gestalt test does not show any serious alterations and no perseveration, except for one "collision" (Figure 4 is practically superimposed on Figure 3); otherwise, the sequence is orderly but the figures are rather small, with little line pressure, like his human figures and HTP drawings.

---

[2] Actually, he has only one AG response, but two Aggressive Contents (AgC) and four Aggressive Past (AgP) responses, which suggest the presence of sadomasochistic elements.

Table 3. Other test data: WAIS

Information	16	Picture completion	5
Comprehension	14	Picture arrangement	11
Arithmetic	14	Block design	14
Similarities	11	Object assembly	10
Digit span	11		
Vocabulary	11	Verbal IQ	116
		Performance IQ	87
		Total IQ	103

Note. WAIS = Wechsler Adult Intelligence Scale.

The story of the DAT (Draw an Animal Test) is rather striking (he drew a male cat):

> The cat lived alone in a house destroyed by the war. His only friend was a mouse with which he decided to live because everything else had disappeared. One day all the food was gone and as a consequence the only one who would survive would be the one who ate the other. But since the cat loved the mouse and the mouse loved the cat, and they knew that the one who ate the other would be most wretched, they decided not to eat each other and died of hunger.

Follow-Up Data

The EEG showed a temporal but not epileptic dysrhythmia in hyperventilation. He was prescribed medical therapy and the second EEG showed almost complete improvement 1 year later. The neurologist supposed its origin to be related either to the scarlet fever at age 4 years, or the rheumatic fever at age 12, which kept Alex in bed for many weeks.

Psychoanalytic treatment was initiated with three weekly sessions, soon prolonged to four on the patient's demand, with rapidly diminished tranquillizer medication.

Alex's second WAIS (Total IQ = 126; Verbal IQ = 126; Performance IQ = 115) and Rorschach were administered by another psychologist nearly 3 years later, with the aim of assessing treatment evolution (2 years; see Appendix B).

The second Rorschach protocol sounded less dramatic, especially on the last three colored cards, showing some very basic changes: the very important inversion of the EB toward introversion, which, with the increase of good *M* responses – even if there are still three negative *M'* responses – and with the disappearance of the passive ideational orientation (now *Ma* > *Mp*), enables Alex to "think more and feel less" primitively (pure *C'* and *Fd* responses are now absent, there are fewer DQv), together with the decrease of depression (DEPI), despite the persistence of morbid thoughts (MOR). Nevertheless, the SCZI and PTI continue to be 6 and 5, respectively. Self-esteem has changed too and his self-image now approaches a more normal range, (H:(H)+Hd+(Hd)), and even if PHR >> GHR, he now has 3 COP, probably is less isolated, less emotionally avoidant (higher *Afr*), and moving toward better affective modulation in spite of the still present, but quite diminished, emotional retention (*C'*); there is also less concern about the body. His narcissism[3] has now come to the fore (see the second structural summary). Therefore, despite these improvements the general impression is still rather negative –mostly due to SCZI and PTI – also shown by the Maladjustment Index (MI). He is now positive on four items only: *WDA%* < .75, *MOR* > 2, *Gh – Ph* < 0, and *WSum6* > 12; in other words, *AdjD* < 0 continues to be negative, as well as *C* > 0 and *EGO* > .33 or > .44. This is to say that the improvement, according to this new index, is centered on the self and the affective sphere.

Follow-Up Data Provided by Alex's Psychoanalyst

Alex's analyst, 8 years after the first assessment (the seventh year of treatment), describes the now 23-year-old patient in the following terms:

> In some aspects Alex has shown a positive evolution. His aggressive fits have disappeared. In general, he has good relations with family and friends. Since he gave up playing rugby, due to a lack of time, he no longer suffers from physical complaints (dislocated shoulder whenever he was tackled too violently).
> Intellectually he is a brilliant student, particularly in higher mathematics (!). But the still persisting problem is his difficulty in relating to women. He has had sexual relations with prostitutes and almost with a slightly older girlfriend (who could not tolerate penetration). Later on, he had several romances that did not last. He is very shy and has great difficulty in expressing

---

[3] I have observed such an emergence more than once after the disappearance or diminution of a severe depression.

affection verbally as well as physically. All of this is related to a more deep-seated problem: his foot fetishism[4].

The attraction to his mother's feet is a memory from the age of 5 or 6, later on followed by masturbation with fantasies in which the woman touched his penis with her feet, and still later that she kicked him with her naked foot. These fantasies continue to exist. Many times, he has become excited looking at girls' feet, and a few times has enacted these fantasies with prostitutes. All of this makes him feel very ashamed and depressed.

Among many, the most useful hypothesis to continue the analytic work was that Alex's fear of harming the woman–mother becomes transformed into masochistic submission to her (see the DAT); when she kicks him, humiliating him, he can have an orgasm. The displacement from the vagina to the foot, apart from the evidently phallic aspect, is linked with the fantasy of perforating and killing the woman with his penis. It is important to keep in mind that the patient's mother has a very pretty face but a monstrous body, due to an enormous and irreducible obesity. She was fat since he was a small child.

Alex is now (5 years after the termination of analysis, which lasted for about 10 years) a brilliant researcher in economics and has returned to work at a prestigious university where he completed his doctoral thesis a few years earlier, in another country. His perversion has disappeared completely [the analyst knew this because Alex entered therapy together with his first wife, and their female therapist, a good friend of Alex's analyst, consulted him about it]. Alex and his first wife did not have sexual difficulties but their relationship was strained because his wife had an exceedingly hysterical character structure. They finally separated and now he is living with a very wonderful woman artist in that other country.

Discussion

This very positive development is rather surprising in view of the unfavorable initial clinical impression and the prognosis derived from the first (and also the second) Rorschach; unfortunately, there was no third and/or last Rorschach. Nevertheless, one cannot lose sight of the fact that Alex's crisis occurred in

---

[4] Very strikingly in his second Rorschach a female shoe and toes appeared as the content of an F− response to Card V (R16) that according to Rausch de Traubenberg and Boizou (1977) refers to the representation of the self.

adolescence, a very difficult age in which the great and central diagnostic difficulty and challenge reside, precisely in distinguishing between a psychotic episode without later collapse and the initiation of a lasting psychotic or schizophrenic breakdown with posterior deterioration.

It should be mentioned too that Alex's psychoanalyst, also a psychiatrist and familiar with the Rorschach test, always maintained that Alex was not schizophrenic, but had a schizoid personality structure. His comment on the continued absence of texture in the second Rorschach was: "That is due to his phobia of close contact."

The second protocol, with the emergence of the narcissistic aspect and one clear borderline merger response (Card VI; see Campo & Vilar, 1990), might suggest a "borderline schizophrenia" (according to Blatt and Auerbach's 1988 conceptualization), and it is also true that in the first Rorschach the defenses are predominantly of the borderline type (Cooper et al., 1988).

However, the SCZI of 6 and the PTI of 5 continue to be at least bothersome. I believe that Alex was neither simulating nor malingering on the first or the second test. Also, I do not know how far the temporal EEG – in hyperventilation – could have co-determined his fit of rage, as well as the high pure C production at the time of the first protocol. In any case it seemed clear that the first Rorschach registered a psychotic episode at that time. In fact, in the second Rorschach the CONTAM has disappeared and the ALOGs have diminished to 1. But still, the rest of his thinking and perception continued to be rather peculiar and distorted despite the quite positive increase in the *XA* and *WDA%'*, while *X*–% remains basically the same.

So, did the Rorschach fail in this case? Or did the two indexes fail? A good question. To begin with, Alex continued therapy and the positive follow-up data tell us that his was a psychotic episode; one more reason to celebrate the change from SCZI to PTI in the CS, and the latter does not stigmatize the subject as the SCZI does.

Regarding the issue of the *M*– responses, in Alex's first protocol the 3 *M*– responses were undoubtedly negative. But in the second one, I would like to reproduce an instance of an *M*– in which the negative quality of the perception was *not* contained in the human figure and movement; this would actually reduce his *M*– to 2. The response was:

I: It could be a headless woman (D4) who is supporting two big animals (D2) with her hands, or two large artificial wings... that woman would be in an excessively symmetrical position, so much so that she appears to be crucified and the two animals she is holding up with her hands look like a mixture of bear with wings (*F-*) or that seem to be, that are... rendering homage like in a cult to the goddess that would be the woman... (W).

Now, regarding the SCZI and its "misdeeds" in Alex's case, does it point erroneously to schizophrenia, or simply to psychosis like the PTI does? This point raises another problem: When is it schizophrenia and when psychosis? This question seems important too since, for instance, in cluster analysis, the positive SCZI or PTI organize the whole interpretative sequence in a certain direction, starting from the cognitive triad, while this may not be the main or only nucleus of the problem, as my interpretative sequence analysis attempted to highlight.

In my experience (see Campo, 1995, Chapter 12 on schizophrenia, or Rovira & Campo, 2007), albeit limited regarding the Rorschach and psychosis, what I think is that – with few exceptions – I do not only rely on the Rorschach alone although I always trust it, and it is my best friend. I always tend to include other tests in an assessment: for example, the projective drawings (e.g., HTPP and DAT), Sentence Completion, the ORT (Object Relations Technique), the Bender, MMPI, and, if needed, the WISC or WAIS, that is, I follow a multimethod approach. Notwithstanding these explanations, I do believe that the Rorschach, apart from being so interesting, rich, and fascinating, always helps me to better understand a person. In addition, it is rarely boring since, like each person, each Rorschach is different.

In my opinion the Rorschach describes a subject's functioning better than many other tests because it operates simultaneously on three levels: conscious, preconscious, and unconscious; cognitively, emotionally, and object-relationally. In the confrontation between the two indexes used in this paper and the whole protocol, I argue that the protocol always wins since it represents the whole person, and it is in this aspect that the Rorschach is so useful and truthful. Indexes alone, with their psychiatric connotation (specifically the SCZI) are too limited to reach a true psychological assessment.

In the last instance, the Rorschach is not a psychiatric instrument like the DSM, and it should not be used in order to provide such a type of diagnosis (a salient aspect emphasized by Exner himself and many other Rorschach authors). Instead, it is much more useful and accurate as an instrument to understand how a person functions, cognitively, dynamically, interpersonally, and only by extension psychiatrically. But this extension does not depend on the Rorschach test, for in essence it depends on the expertise of the clinical psychologist who uses the Rorschach, on his/her theoretical and psychopathological orientation (that may be very varied), and primarily on the interest to understand and help patients.

References

Blatt, S. J., & Auerbach, J. S. (1988). Tres tipos de pacientes borderline y sus Respuestas diferenciales a tests psicológicos [Three types of borderline patients and their differential responses to psychological tests]. *Revista de la Sociedad Española del Rorschach y Métodos Proyectivos (SERYMP), 1*, 27–38.

Campo, V. (1979). On the meaning of the inanimate movement response (m). *British Journal of Projective Psychology and Personality Study, 24*(1–2), 1–6, 1–19.

Campo, V. (1993). An old friend revisited: In the throes of the SCZI index. *British Journal of Projective Psychology, 38*(1), 2–28.

Campo, V. (1995). *Estudios clínicos con el Rorschach en niños, adolescentes y adultos* [Clinical studies with the Rorschach in children, adolescents and adults]. Barcelona, Spain: Paidós y Fundación Vidal i Barraquer.

Campo, V. (2003–2004). Múltiples color-sombreado: ¿Todos tienen el mismo significado? [Color-shading blends: Do all of them have the same meaning?]. *Revista de la SERYMP, 16–17*, 83–96.

Campo, V. (2000). The SCZI index and the normative sample of Barcelona (1993). *Rorschachiana, 24*, 28–38. https://doi.org/10.1027/1192-5604.24.1.28

Campo, V. (2015, August). *The M-problem*. Paper presented at the CSIRA Congress, Milan, Italy.

Campo, V., & Vilar, N. (1990). Acerca de los contenidos, defensas y relaciones objetales borderline [On borderline contents, defences and object relations]. *Revista de la Sociedad Española del Rorschach y Métodos Proyectivos (SERYMP), 3*, 28–32.

Campo, V., & Vilar, N. (2007). Rorschach Comprehensive System data for a sample of 517 adults from Spain (Barcelona). *Journal of Personality Assessment, 89*, S149–S153. https://doi.org/10.1080/00223890701583432

Cooper, S. H., Perry, J. C., & Arnow, D. (1988). An empirical approach to the study of defense mechanisms: 1. Reliability and preliminary validity of the Rorschach Defense Scales. *Journal of Personality Assessment, 52*, 187–203.

Exner, J. E. (1990, April). *1990 alumni newsletter*. Asheville, NC: Rorschach Workshops.

Exner, J. E. (1997–2003). *The Rorschach: A comprehensive system. Vol. I: Basic foundations and principles of interpretation* (4th ed.). Hoboken, NJ: John Wiley & Sons.

Exner, J. E., & Erdberg, P. (2005–2007). *The Rorschach: A comprehensive system. Advanced interpretation* (3rd ed.). Hoboken, NJ: Wiley.

Gacono, C. B., & Meloy, J. R. (1994). *The Rorschach assessment of aggressive and psychopathic personalities*. Hillsdale, NJ: Erlbaum.

Kalla, O., Wahlstrom, J., Aaltonen, J., Holma, J., Tuimala, P., & Mattlar, C.-E. (2002). Cognitive deficits in patients with first-episode psychosis as identified by Exner's Schizophrenia Index in Finland and Spain. *Rorschachiana, 25*, 175–194. https://doi.org/10.1027/1192-5604.25.1.175

Phillipson, H. (1995). *The object relations technique*. London, UK: Tavistock Publications.

Rausch de Traubenberg, N., & Boizou, N. F. (1977). *Le Rorschach en Clinique Infantile, l'imaginaire et la réelle chez l'enfant* [The Rorschach in clinical work with children, the imaginary and the real childhood]. Paris, France: Dunod.

Rovira, F., & Campo, V. (2007). El avestruz que no ve el mundo. Desarrollo de un trastorno psicótico infantil. Seguimiento con dibujos y Rorschach [The ostrich that does not see the world. Development of an infantile psychotic disturbance. Follow up with drawings and the Rorschach]. *Revista de la Sociedad Española del Rorschach y Métodos Proyectivos, 20*, 53–72.

Smith, S. R., Baity, M. R., Knowles, E. S., & Hilsenroth, M. J. (2001). Assessment of disordered thinking in children and adolescents: The Rorschach perceptual-thinking index. *Journal of Personality Assessment, 77*(3), 447–463. https://doi.org/10.1207/S15327752JPA7703_06

Received February 10, 2015
Revision received August 25, 2017
Accepted September 22, 2017
Published online May 9, 2018

Vera Campo
Sociedad Catalana del Rorschach y Métodos Proyectivos (SCRIMP)
Barcelona
Spain
veracampo@gmail.com

Appendix A

Rorschach (translated from Spanish)[1]

I

1. A butterfly, a folded paper (refers to the technique of making the blots), a photo in white and black, something immovable, motionless. Pretty, balanced colors. It expresses some thought, something that flies...

2. Blood between two pieces of glass, dry blood.

3. Viruses in...cancer.

4. Clouds in the shape of airplanes or birds...something bilateral. Nothing more.

II

5. Something bilateral...blood, striking.

6. Beetle (peers closely at D6).

7. Clouds with blood.

E. Repeats R (This formula will not be repeated)

1. The whole, wings, body, a butterfly of death because it is of black color, the same on both sides, dead, shattered because it's splattered, or looks like a bat too because once I saw a dead one. E: You said it is immovable? S: Because it's dead. E: And pretty colors? Gray, white, few colors E: Expressing some thought? S: Something violent like death, because it is a butterfly and the shape of the wings.

2. The whole, because of the stains (points to shading) and because it looks compressed, at some time it had the color of blood but it already has the color of death, inorganic...

3. Small black things, something that expands as a sign of illness, to the left black places that are growing in size, there are more viruses...(W).

4. The whole, it has the shape more of a bird, the color and the shape, like flying between the white and the nothingness of the sky, something lost in the infinity of space (points to S around blot). E: Clouds? S: heavy storm clouds.

5. All of it (but also points to D3) stained, by the black and the red which is equivalent to imminent death

6. (WS)Because of the way it ends up front (D4), this (S) a void, wider, a bit fat, and blood (D2+D3) it is eating from the man. The faces of death too, sadistic color, wanting to hurt others (refers to R 10).

7. The whole, after a storm when the sun comes out or there is lightning, it's more striking, not so gay, black and red.

---

[1] It was quite difficult to translate this protocol from Spanish into English because of the enigmatic language, but also to code it. In addition, in Gacono and Meloy's (1994) aggression scores were included the coding: AgC = Content and AgPast.

(Continued on next page)

(Continued)

8. The bones of a person, an operation.	8. (WS) The way it's open (S) and the bones and spilled blood, the spine and the black, rather inorganic tissues, rather dead already because of the shape, the barrenness, a bit loathsome (points to dark lines in D6) in the bloody part.
9. A bat. A bit of something living...real...a work of art...hm...	9. Once I saw a dead one, the face (D4), shattered like this because of the flat shape and the blood. E: You said something living? S: Which is the blood, a blot like that which manifests itself, it looks like a brushstroke rather similar to the artist's thought, which is to kill or commit suicide because of the shape of the body opened in the middle and the color.
10. Up here two faces of blood and down here two apes fighting and blood on them. Not two people fighting, but who make others fight in their stead. Nothing more.	10. They would be globules (D2), inside parts that also have their personality, the blood gives the sensation of life and of death. Human faces, a bit deformed because of the flattened lines, with blood pressure in the veins, not very expressive. Up here (D2) organizers of the struggle with mental force and down here with the brute force of the body. They look more like gorillas (refers to the apes in D6). (W)

III

11. Two persons dancing...thoughts of blood, faces like foxes. Dancing something, the same thing, with the same movements, a table in the middle. Nothing more.	11. (W) A dance due more to the folded paper, an old dance, of 1900, because of the antique suits no longer fashionable, the black color. I thought of a man and a woman because of the elevation there (bust) and with the face of a crow or fox. There is blood right besides their heads, apparently friendly thoughts but at bottom they hate each other, and something that separates them a little (points to D3). One can see what they think (D2) and don't say.

IV

12. A dead animal, a dead bat, turned into rock, hm...face down with spread legs. Two spread arms, hm...	12. (W) What was the skin, which is already almost nonliving matter, because of the color and the lack of movement, skin and bones, the head up here (D3), that like the hands (D4) and the continuation of the body, like shattered on the ground and it doesn't show its face...

(Continued on next page)

(Continued)

13. Very barren, lacking life, a hell, gooseflesh...	13. (W) Looks like what a man could think when things go badly, black thoughts because black is a color neither strong nor...always the same. E: You said barren? S: A sandy surface, always the same, eroded relief like mountains (points to shading), more than seen, imagined. E: Gooseflesh? S: Because of the edge (points to contours).
14. A toad...	14. The whole, the shape, head, legs, tail.
15. An X-ray of the spine.	15. (D5) Because of the black color.
V	
16. A butterfly.	16. (W) It has the shape, more compact, and though it's in death it doesn't look so eroded by exterior agents, because of the contrast with the white it looks as it were flying but at the same time still.
17. Two people pressed[2], one on top of the other. E: Pardon? S: Pressed (shows location on Card).	17. (W) Resting on, two men or two women, they are the same, the legs (D10), arms (D9), breasts (lower part of Dd35) and here a bit like horns (D6). E: Horns? S: Yes...
18. A divided bull, split in half, losing everything, everything escaping it, something flying...and dead.	18. (W) Bull because of the horns and legs and everything, the stomach is dissolving, disassembling at the sides.
19. The cranium split in half. Nothing more.	19. (Dd99) The central line, only the line that divides the hemispheres, because they would not be thinking, not very gay, it is something that is true but that they don't like.
VI	
20. A crucified Christ.	20. The whole, the face, arms, legs, the human mixed up with the immaterial because of the size (points to D1).
21. Something between two pieces of glass split in half, something ex-human.	21. (W) Always the flattened shape, the perimeter seems to be the product of the squashing; once it was human but it isn't any longer.
22. Bones...disintegrating bones. Something dead face down.	22. (W) The shape of the center and the white (Dd32) look like bones that are merging with minerals, because of the color and the hues of the whole... rather face up if it is a Christ...
23. An X-ray with mustaches. Something opened up down the middle, a strange photo. Nothing more.	23. (W) Part of an X-ray, the rest de decayed by time, because of the edges. E: Mustaches? S: It could be an X-ray of a man or a cat. E: How would that be? S: A man converted into a cat, split.

[2] Translation note: Peculiar and erroneous use of the word in Spanish, corrected in the inquiry by a word of similar sound: *apurados-apoyados*.

(Continued on next page)

(Continued)

VII

24. Two faces looking at each other.

25. A harbor, no ship…high mountains… desert of men, without men, animals or plants, with minerals and water (DS7), without water too. Something without life. Nothing more.

VIII

26. Two lions climbing a mountain.

27. A parasol…pretty colors, watery, warm…bi-lateral.

28. A colored skeleton and held up by wires…something progressive[3], progressive change of colors, beginning of the world. Nothing more.

IX

29. Someone eating, skin, blood, with a fork, two noses with green blood and pink tongue, a wall in the middle. The colors are very expressive in the center and become lighter towards the sides. A mental thought, the middle, a glass in the middle, a surrealist picture. Nothing more.

X

30. Painter of walls, gayety, little animals, there is always a dividing line.
31. Tentacles.
32. Two little babies.
33. Looks like the color of skin.
34. Renewed blood. Nothing more.

24. (W) (two faces on whole inner contours). Faces of men, the forehead, nose, the expression is a bit dead, without much expression.

25. (WS) The water is the white, specially because of the color and the water is all white, there isn't much difference…

26. (W) They try to climb but can't yet…many geological ages because the colors are different (D6), they are about to fall…

27. (Ddo99 = D4 + whole central line). Of a forest, because it has the shape of a tree, a pine tree and the color too.

28. (D6) Colored vertebrae, the animals not so much, the central part, vertebrae and spine.

29. (W) The noses (Dd28), the blood (D6), the forks (Dd21) and the wall (D5), they are men with the mouth a bit covered and one can't see the eyes and blood streaming up here (D3) because here would be the forehead and there the thoughts come out (Dd34) because it is narrow and square with the color of blood (Dd34) because it is narrow and square with the blood and skin.

30. The whole, loud colors, many colors.
31. (D1) Of an octopus or…or spiders, more like an octopus.
32. (D2) Yellow color because they have light complexions, the face and the body.
33. (D15) Yellow skin.
34. (D9) Pink, because it is rather lively, strong red.

[3] Translation note: Progressive in the sense of liberal, new idea.

(Continued on next page)

(Continued)

TEST DATE:			GRP: 2		CAT: 2	ID: 0	FILE:563
NAME: ALEX			AGE: 15		SEX: M	MS: Single	ED: 9

SEQUENCE OF SCORES

CARD	NO	LOC	#	DETERMINANT(S)	(2)	CONTENT(S)	POP Z	SPECIAL SCORES
I	1	WSo	1	FC'o		A	3.5	ALOG,MOR,AgPast
	2	Wv	1	Y		Bl		MOR
	3	Wv	1	C'F.ma–		Id		MOR,AgC
	4	WS+	1	FC'.FMao		A,Cl	3.5	CON
II	5	Wv	1	C.C'		Bl		ALOG,MOR,AB
	6	WS+	1	FMa.CF–		A,Bl	4.5	FAB,oral
	7	Wv	1	C'.C		Cl,Bl		FAB2
	8	WS+	1	FC'.CF–		An,Bl	4.5	MOR,AgPast
	9	W+	1	CF–		A,Bl,Art	4.5	MOR,DR,AgPast
	10	W+	1	Ma.FMa.CF–	2	Hd,A,Bl	4.5	INC2,AG,PHR
III	11	W+	1	Ma.C.FC'o		H,Bl,Hx,Cg	P 5.5	COP,INC2,FAB2,ALOG,PHR
IV	12	Wo	1	FC'u		A	2.0	MOR,DV,AgPast
	13	Wv	1	Mp.C'.V		Hx		AB,MOR,PHR
	14	Wo	1	Fu		A	2.0	INC
	15	Do	5	FC'o		Xy		
V	16	Wo	1	Fo		A	P 1.0	DR
	17	W+	1	Mpo	2	H	2.5	DV,INC,PHR
	18	Wo	1	mp–		A	1.0	MOR,AgPast
	19	Ddo	99	F–		An		MOR,DR
VI	20	Wo	1	F–		(H)	2.5	MOR,ALOG,PHR,AgPast
	21	Wv	1	Fu		Id		MOR,DV,AgPast
	22	Wv	1	YF–		An		MOR
	23	Wo	1	F–		Xy,Ad	2.5	INC2,MOR
VII	24	W+	1	Mp–	2	Hd	2.5	PHR
	25	WS/	1	C'Fo		Na	4.0	INC

(Continued on next page)

(Continued)

VIII	26	W+	1	FMa.CFo	2	A,Ls	P 4.5	AgC
	27	Ddo	99	FCu		Bt		ALOG
	28	Do	6	FC−		An		MOR,INC,DV
IX	29	W+	1	Mp.CF.mp−	2	Art,Hd,Bl,Fd	5.5	DR,FAB2,PHR,oral
X	30	Wv	1	C		Art		
	31	Do	1	Fo		A		
	32	Do	2	FC−	2	H		ALOG,INC,PHR?
	33	Dv	15	C		Id		
	34	Dv	9	C		Bl		

SUMMARY OF APPROACH

I:WSo.Wv.Wv.WS+
II:Wv.WS+.Wv.WS+.W+.W+
III:W+
IV:Wo.Wv.Wo.Do
V:Wo.W+.Wo.Ddo
VI:Wo.Wv.Wv.Wo
VII:W+.WS/
VIII:W+.Ddo.Do
IX:W+
X:Wv.Do.Do.Dv.Dv

STRUCTURAL SUMMARY

LOCATION FEATURES	DETERMINANTS		CONTENTS	S-CONSTELLATION
	BLENDS	SINGLE		
				NO..FV+VF+V+FD>2
			H = 3	YES..Col-Shd Bl>0
	C'F.m	M = 2	(H) = 1	YES..Ego<.31,>.44
Zf = 18	FC'.FM	FM = 0	Hd = 3	YES..MOR > 3
ZSum = 60.5	C.C'	m = 1	(Hd) = 0	NO..Zd > +− 3.5
ZEst = 59.5	FM.CF	FC = 3	Hx = 2	NO..es > EA
	C'.C	CF = 1	A = 11	YES..CF+C > FC
W = 26	FC'.CF	C = 3	(A) = 0	YES..X+% < .70
D = 6	M.FM.CF	Cn = 0	Ad = 1	YES..S > 3
W+D = 32	M.C.FC'	FC' = 3	(Ad) = 0	NO..P < 3 or > 8
Dd = 2	M.C'.V	C'F = 1	An = 4	NO..Pure H < 2
S = 5	FM.CF	C' = 0	Art = 3	NO..R < 17
	M.CF.m	FT = 0	Ay = 0	6.....TOTAL
DQ		TF = 0	Bl = 10	SPECIAL SCORES
+ = 10		T = 0	Bt = 1	Lv1 Lv2
o = 13		FV = 0	Cg = 1	DV = 4x1 0x2

(Continued on next page)

(Continued)

v/+ = 1	VF = 0	Cl = 2	INC = 5x2	3x4
v = 10	V = 0	Ex = 0	DR = 4x3	0x6
	FY = 0	Fd = 1	FAB = 1x4	3x7
	YF = 1	Fi = 0	ALOG = 6x5	
	Y = 1	Ge = 0	CON = 1x7	
FORM QUALITY	Fr = 0	Hh = 0	Raw Sum6 = 27	
FQx MQual W+D	rF = 0	Ls = 1	Wgtd Sum6 = 100	
+ = 0 = 0 = 0	FD = 0	Na = 1		
o = 9 = 2 = 9	F = 7	Sc = 0	AB = 2	GHR = 0
u = 4 = 0 = 3		Sx = 0	AG = 1	PHR = 8
− = 14 = 3 = 13		Xy = 2	COP = 1	MOR = 15
none = 7 = 1 = 7		Id = 3	CP = 0	PER = 0
	(2) = 6		PSV = 0	

RATIOS, PERCENTAGES, AND DERIVATIONS

R = 34	L = 0.26		FC:CF+C = 3:12	COP = 1 AG = 1
			Pure C = 6	GHR:PHR = 0: 8
EB = 6:16.5	EA = 22.5	EBPer = 2.8	SumC':WSumC = 11:16.5	a:p = 7: 6
eb = 7:14	es = 21	D = 0	Afr = 0.36	Food = 1
	Adj es = 18	Adj D = +1	S = 5	SumT = 0
			Blends:R = 11:34	Hum Cont = 7
FM = 4	C' = 11	T = 0	CP = 0	Pure H = 3
m = 3	V = 1	Y = 2		PER = 0
				Iso Indx = 0.24
a:p = 7: 6	Sum6 = 27	XA% = 0.38	Zf = 18.0	3r+(2)/R = 0.18
Ma:Mp = 2: 4	Lv2 = 6	WDA% = 0.38	W:D:Dd = 26: 6: 2	Fr+rF = 0
2AB+Art+Ay = 7	WSum6 = 100	X−% = 0.41	W:M = 26: 6	SumV = 1
MOR =15	M− = 3	S− = 2	Zd = +1.0	FD = 0
	Mnone = 1	Xu% = 0.12	PSV = 0	An+Xy = 6
		X+% = 0.26	DQ+ = 10	MOR = 15
		Xu% = 0.12	DQv = 10	H:(H)Hd(Hd) = 3: 4
PTI = 5*	DEPI = 7*	CDI = 3	S-CON = 6	HVI = YES OBS = No

CONSTELLATIONS TABLE

PTI (Perceptual-Thinking Index):
YES...(XA% < .70) AND (WDA% < .75)
YES...(X−% >.29)
YES...(Sum Level 2 > 2) AND (FAB2 > 0)

SCZI (Schizophrenia Index)
YES...Either X+ < .61 and S−%
        < .41 or X+% < .50
YES...X−% > .29

(Continued on next page)

(Continued)

YES...EITHER: (R < 17) AND (WSUM6 > 12)
   OR...: (R > 16) AND (WSUM6 > 17)
YES...EITHER: (M− > 1)
   OR...: (X−% > .40)

DEPI (DEPRESSION INDEX):
Positive if 5 or more conditions are true:
YES...(FV+VF+V > 0) OR (FD > 2)
YES...(Col-Shd Blends > 0) OR (S > 2)
YES...(3r+(2)/R > .50* and Fr+rF = 0)
   OR (3r+(2)/R < .33)
YES...(Afr < .46* OR (Blends < 4)
YES...(SumShading > FM+m) OR
   (SumC' > 2)
YES...(MOR > 2) OR (2AB+(Art+Ay) > 3)
YES...(COP < 2) OR (Isolate/R > .24)

HV (HYPERVIGILANCE INDEX):
Positive if Condition 1 is true and at least 4 of the others are true.

YES...(1) FT+TF+T = 0
- - - - - - - -
YES...(2) Zf > 12
No...(3) Zd > +3.5
YES...(4) S > 3
YES...(5) H+(H)+Hd+(Hd) > 6
No...(6) (H)+(A)+(Hd)+(Ad) > 3
YES...(7) H+A:Hd+Ad < 4:1
No...(8) Cg > 3

YES...Either FQ >= FQu or FQ−
   > FQo + FQ+
*YES...Sum L2 Sp. Sc. > and
   FAB2 > 9
YES...Either RawSUM6 > 6 or
   WSUM6 > 17
YES...Either M− > 1 or X−%
   > .40

CDI (COPING DEFICIT INDEX):
Positive if 4 or 5 conditions are true:
No...(EA < 6) OR (AdjD < 0)
YES...(COP < 2) AND (AG < 2)
YES...(WSumC < 2.5) OR (Afr< .46)
No...(Passive > Active+1) OR
   (Pure H < 2)
YES...(Sum T > 1) OR
   (Isolate/R > .24) OR (Food > 0)

OBS (OBSESSIVE STYLE INDEX):

No...(1) Dd > 3
YES...(2) Zf > 12
No...(3) Zd > +3.0
No...(4) Populars > 7
No...(5) FQ+ > 1
- - - - - - - -
Positive if one or more is true:
No...Conditions 1 to 5
   Are All True
No...2 or more of 1 to 4
   are true AND FQ+ > 3
No...3 or more of 1 to 5
   are true AND X+% > .89
No...FQ+ > 3 AND X+% > .89

*--Corrected for age norms.
Note. From Exner (1997–2003).

Appendix B

Second Structural Summary

TEST DATE:	GRP: 1	CAT: 2	ID:563	FILE:563.2
NAME: ALEX	Second Rorschach	AGE: 18 SEX:M	RACE: MS:Single	ED:12

STRUCTURAL SUMMARY

LOCATION FEATURES	DETERMINANTS BLENDS	SINGLE	CONTENTS	S-CONSTELLATION
				NO..FV+VF+V+FD>2
			H = 8	YES..Col-Shd Bl>0
Zf = 27	M.CF.m.FV	M = 8	(H) = 1	YES..Ego<.31,>.44
ZSum = 96.5	CF.m.Fr	FM = 1	Hd = 5	YES..MOR > 3
ZEst = 91.5	M.FC.FM	m = 0	(Hd) = 1	YES..Zd > +− 3.5
	m.FC'	FC = 1	Hx = 0	NO..es > EA
W = 26	m.C'F	CF = 2	A = 16	YES..CF+C > FC
D = 5	FM.CF	C = 0	(A) = 0	YES..X+% < .70
W+D = 31	FC.m	Cn = 0	Ad = 2	YES..S > 3
Dd = 5	FM.FV	FC' = 2	(Ad) = 0	NO..P < 3 or > 8
S = 5	FC.FY	C'F = 0	An = 1	NO..Pure H < 2
	CF.FM	C' = 0	Art = 5	NO..R < 17
		FT = 0	Ay = 0	7.....TOTAL SPECIAL SCORES
DQ		TF = 0	Bl = 3	Lv1 Lv2
+ = 15		T = 0	Bt = 2	DV = 0x1 0x2
o = 17		FV = 0	Cg = 2	INC = 7x2 7x4
v/+ = 0		VF = 0	Cl = 0	DR = 10x3 0x6
v = 4		V = 0	Ex = 0	FAB = 1x4 3x7
		FY = 0	Fd = 0	ALOG = 1x5
		YF = 0	Fi = 1	CON = 0x7
		Y = 0	Ge = 1	Raw Sum6 = 29

(Continued on next page)

(Continued)

	FORM QUALITY			Fr = 0	Hh = 0		Wgtd Sum6 =102	
	FQx	MQual	W+D	rF = 0	Ls = 1			
+	= 0	= 0	= 0	FD = 0	Na = 0			
o	= 11	= 4	= 10	F =12	Sc = 1		AB = 1	GHR = 1
u	= 9	= 3	= 9		Sx = 1		AG = 1	PHR = 15
−	= 16	= 3	= 12		Xy = 1		COP = 3	MOR = 11
none	= 0	= 0	= 0		Id = 3		CP = 0	PER = 0
				(2) =15				PSV = 0

RATIOS, PERCENTAGES, AND DERIVATIONS

R = 36		L = 0.50			FC:CF+C	= 4: 6	COP = 3 AG = 1	
EB = 10: 8.0		EA = 18.0	EBPer = N/A		SumC':WSumC	= 4: 8.0	GHR:PHR	= 1:15
eb = 10: 7		es = 17		D = 0	Afr	= 0.44	a:p	= 11: 9
		Adj es = 13		Adj D = +1	S = 5		Food	= 0
					Blends:R	= 10:36	SumT	= 0
FM = 5		C' = 4	T = 0		CP	= 0	Hum Cont	= 15
m = 5		V = 2	Y = 1				Pure H	= 8
							PER	= 0
							Iso Indx	= 0.11
a:p	= 11: 9	Sum6	= 29	XA% = 0.56	Zf	= 27.0	3r+(2)/R	= 0.50
Ma:Mp	= 7: 3	Lv2	= 10	WDA% = 0.61	W:D:Dd	= 26: 5: 5	Fr+rF	= 1
2AB+Art+Ay	= 7	WSum6	= 102	X−% = 0.44	W:M	= 26:10	SumV	= 2
MOR	= 11	M−	= 3	S− = 4	Zd	= +5.0	FD	= 0
		Mnone	= 0	P = 5	PSV	= 0	An+Xy	= 2
				X+% = 0.31	DQ+	= 15	MOR	=11
				Xu% = 0.25	DQv	= 4	H:(H)Hd(Hd)	= 8: 7
PTI = 5*		DEPI = 5*		CDI = 1	S-CON	= 7	HVI =YES OBS = No	

Summary

The aim of this partial follow-up study (first Rorschach in pretherapy assessment, second Rorschach after 2 years of psychoanalytic treatment) is to illustrate and discuss a very difficult and interesting to code Rorschach protocol of a 15-year-old adolescent who, in a fit of rage, beat up his family, and whose clinical evolution was very positive after 10 years of psychoanalysis. The study also aims to show the usefulness of the Rorschach in order to better understand not only the performance (following R/PAS) during test administration, but the usefulness of knowing more about the richness of a subject's inner world and object relations. The discussion turns to the use of two Comprehensive System (CS) indices – the SCZI and PTI in favor of the latter, despite the fact that both indices continued to be 6 and 5 in the two protocols (even if in the second Rorschach positive changes were evident in emotional and ideational aspects). The importance and implication of $M-$ responses are also included in the discussion.

Résumé

Le but de cette étude partielle sur une suite thérapeutique (premièrement, le Rorschach comme évaluation pre-therapie, deuxièmement, le Rorschach après deux ans de psychanalyse) est d'illustrer et discuter d'un protocole du Rorschach difficile à coder d'un adolescent de 15 ans, qui dans un accès de rage donne des coups à toute sa famille. Après 10 ans de psychanalyse, son évolution clinique a été très positive. De même, cette étude essaie de démontrer l'utilité du Rorschach pour mieux comprendre; non seulement la *performance* (dans le sens de l'R/PAS) pendant l'administration du test, mais aussi la richesse du monde interne et des relations à l'object du sujet. La discussion tourne autour de l'utilisation de deux indices du Système Intégré d'Exner: SCZI ou PTI, les données vont en faveur de ce dernier malgré le fait que ces deux facteurs continuent à être 6 et 5 dans les deux protocoles; même si dans le second Rorschach, des changements positifs étaient évidents dans des aspects émotionnels et idéatoires. L'importance et implications des réponses $M-$ sont aussi incluses.

Resumen

La meta de este estudio parcial de un seguimiento (primer Rorschach como evaluación preterapéutica, segundo Rorschach después de dos años de tratamiento psicoanalítico) es la de ilustrar y discutir un muy interesante protocolo de Rorschach, difícil de codificar, de un adolescente de 15 años que en un acceso de furia pegó a toda su familia; después de 10 años de psicoanálisis su evolución clínica posterior fue muy positiva. Asimismo este estudio intenta mostrar la utilidad del Rorschach para comprender mejor no solo la *performance* (en el sentido del R/PAS) durante la administración del test, sino la riqueza del mundo interno y relaciones objetales del sujeto. La discusión gira alrededor del uso de dos índices del Sistema Comprehensivo (SC): SCZI y PTI -y a favor de este último-, a pesar del hecho que ambos continuaron en 6 y 5 en los dos protocolos; aun cuando en el segundo Rorschach se evidenciaron cambios positivos en aspectos emocionales e ideacionales. También se incluye la importancia e implicaciones de las respuestas $M-$.

要約

SCZIかPTIか——統合失調症か精神病か？：ある追跡調査

　　この部分的な追跡調査（最初はセラピーに入る前のロールシャッハ法施行、2回目は2年にわたる精神分析的治療の後のロールシャッハ法施行）の目的は、大変難しいが同時に興味深い15歳の思春期少年のロールシャッハプロトコルのコード化を示し、それを考察することである。その少年はひどくかっとしやすく、家族を痛めつけていたが、10年にわたる精神分析の後の臨床的評価はとても肯定的であった。本研究はまた、検査施行中の遂行（R－PASによる）をよりよく理解するだけでなく、被検者の内的世界と対象関係の豊かさについてより理解することの有用性を示すことである。考察においては、2つの包括システムの指標——SCZIとPTIに焦点が当てられた。2つのプロトコル（2回目のロールシャッハでは、情緒と観念活動の側面に肯定的な変化が明らかであったが）でこの二つの指標は6と5と両方とも継続して該当していた。M－反応の重要性とそこに含まれる意味が、またこの考察に含まれている。

Erratum

Correction to Vari et al., 2017

(https://doi.org/10.1027/1192-5604/a000092)

Article "Investigating Personality and Psychopathology in Patients With Psoriasis" by Chiara Vari et al. (*Rorschachiana*, 2, 2017) contained incorrect affiliations.

The corrected affiliations read as follows:

Alessandro Crisi
Sapienza University of Rome, Italy
Istituto Italiano Wartegg, Italy

Silvana Carlesimo
Istituto Italiano Wartegg, Italy

Antonio G. Richetta
Department of Dermatology and Venereology, Policlinico Umberto I,
Sapienza University of Rome, Italy

The authors and editors regret any inconvenience or confusion this error may have caused.

Reference

Vari, C., Velotti, P., Crisi, A., Carlesimo, S., Richetta, A. G., & Zavattini, G. C. (2017). Investigating personality and psychopathology in patients with psoriasis. *Rorschachiana, 2*, 87–107. https://doi.org/10.1027/1192-5604/a000092

Published online May 9, 2018

Obituary

Vera Campo, 1927–2018

Vera Campo passed away in Barcelona on April 14, 2018.

She was born in Paris in 1927. In her childhood she lived in Hamburg, Copenhagen, and Barcelona, before arriving in Buenos Aires. She studied in the United States, then continued her training as a psychoanalyst in Argentina, and later received her doctorate in Psychology at the University of Barcelona (1986).

She was president of the Argentine Society of Rorschach, and founder of the Spanish Society (of which she was editor of its magazine until the end of her life), and was also a founding partner of the Catalan Society of Rorschach and Projective Methods, which she also presided.

Since her arrival in Barcelona in 1972, she developed an intense teaching, research, and diagnostic work. She always surprised us by her inexhaustible ability to work on the subjects she was passionate about, among them the Rorschach. She dedicated her life to studying, teaching, and divulging her ideas – and participated actively in all the international meetings of the International Society of Rorschach and Projective Methods since 1961 (Freiburg).

She was an active and key member of the Catalan Society of Rorschach and Projective Methods, forming generations of people interested in learning the Rorschach Test as a valuable tool for diagnosis and personality research. She published, in addition to multiple articles in different magazines, three books: *Los niños y el Rorschach* (Children and the Rorschach), *Rorschach en niños, adolescentes y adults* (The Rorschach Test in Children, Adolescents, and Adults), and *Toda una vida con Rorschach* (A Lifetime With the Rorschach).

Her desire to transmit her knowledge and experience led her to other European cities (London, Rome, Helsinki, Vienna ...) to give courses for specialists in the field.

She was a long-standing member of Rorschachiana's Editorial Board. Vera Campo's outstanding contributions included many articles for the journal as well as being a sharp and meticulous reviewer.

She will be greatly missed by the Rorschach community.

Published online May 9, 2018

Research Article

A Normative Study in England With the Rorschach Comprehensive System

Kari Carstairs[1], Sarah Hartley[2], Andrew Peden[3], Justine McCarthy Woods[4], Andre van Graan[5], Anne Andronikof[6], and Patrick Fontan[7]

[1]Carstairs Psychological Associates Limited, Bromley, Kent, UK
[2]Psychologie (UK) Limited, Seaford, East Sussex, UK
[3]St Luke's Centre, Manchester, UK
[4]Adolescent and Young Adult Service, Tavistock Centre, London, UK
[5]Department of Clinical and Experimental Epilepsy, UCL Institute of Neurology, Queens Square, London, UK
[6]Laboratoire IPSé, Université Paris Ouest, Nanterre, France
[7]Circonscription Saint Denis 1, Paris, France

Abstract: This study provides Rorschach data for 88 adults aged 18–65 years from the general population in England. The sample was matched as closely as possible with census data on the variables of gender, age, marital status, ethnicity, geographical location, occupation, and level of education. The Rorschach was administered according to the Comprehensive System by five experienced psychologists. Participants also completed a measure of psychological distress called the CORE. Interscorer reliability was found to be excellent for all variables apart from the six cognitive special scores, for which it was fair. Rorschach data are presented for Comprehensive System variables and compared with Exner's (2007) sample of 450 nonpatient adults in the United States and with the international reference sample (Meyer, Erdberg, & Shaffer, 2007).

Keywords: Comprehensive System, England, normative study, Rorschach

The Rorschach Comprehensive System (Exner, 2003) is founded upon a large amount of normative data. The original norms were based on data from North America. Since their publication, international normative studies involving almost 9,000 participants have been conducted in 17 different countries in Asia, Europe, the Middle East, North and South America, and in Australia. Data for the different international samples differ from the US normative data in some respects. The participants were all nonpatients and results were collated to form the International Reference Sample (Meyer, Erdberg, & Shaffer, 2007). Until the present study, there have been no normative data from England.

The objective of this study was to gather a sample of data from adults of working age in the general population in England in order to determine whether the results differ significantly as compared with the US norms. Such a difference would imply that the clinician should not rely on the US norms and that data for an English sample should be consulted when interpreting Comprehensive System Rorschach results for English examinees.

Method

Five qualified and experienced clinical psychologists were recruited to assess adults from the general population in England with the Rorschach using the Comprehensive System. All examiners were doctoral-level clinical psychologists registered with the Health & Care Professions Council and all were in practice in England for a minimum of 12 years prior to participation in the study. Participants were aged between 18 and 65 years. Every effort was made to gather a sample that was representative of the general population according to the 2011 Office for National Statistics Census data on the variables of gender, marital status, age, ethnicity, level of education, occupation, and geographical region.

Participants were recruited by the examiners using local contacts. Examiners did not test anyone whom they knew personally. Participants were paid £10 for their time; examiners were not reimbursed. The total number of participants assessed by each examiner ranged from 12 to 20 (with one psychologist testing 12 people, one testing 17 people, one testing 19 people, and two testing 20 people), with a total of 88 participants. Data collection began in 2014 and was completed in 2016. There was an introductory session with the team of examiners before data collection to review the informed consent procedure, the criteria for the selection of participants, and the administration of all of the materials so to ensure homogeneity. Participation in the study was estimated to take about 1 hr. Participants were informed that they would not receive any interpretation of their responses. They were advised that confidentiality would be maintained and the results would be communicated by amalgamating their data with data from all of the participants so that results would be reported for the group as a whole but no individual responses would be revealed. Examiners continued to meet regularly and consulted with each other throughout the duration of the research project.

In addition to completing the Rorschach, participants filled out a sheet with questions relating to the demographic variables. All participants were born in the UK, apart from one person who was born on a British Army base in Germany and whose family moved back to the UK when she was a few months old.

Participants were excluded if they: (a) reported having suffered a head injury resulting in unconsciousness; (b) reported having received a diagnosis of a learning disability; (c) presented with any obvious hearing, language, or visual impairments that could interfere with test administration; (d) or reported having had a psychiatric in-patient admission within the preceding 12 months.

Three volunteers were excluded due to a history of head injury that had resulted in a period of unconsciousness. None of the volunteers reported having received a diagnosis of learning disability. One participant mentioned during the administration of the Rorschach that she was color blind, but we decided to retain her results because in responding to the area D5 on card VIII she remarked, "I am color blind but this looks green." None of the volunteers reported having had a psychiatric in-patient admission in the preceding year. Participants were also asked if they considered that they had any kind of disability: one mentioned tinnitus, one mentioned spondylitis, and a third mentioned dyslexia. The remaining 85 participants reported that they did not have any disability.

Participants were also asked if they were taking medication of any kind; 12 participants responded affirmatively. Of these, five indicated that they were taking some kind of antidepressant medication (Prozac, sertraline, and fluoxetine were listed). The remaining seven participants listed statins, antacid medication, the contraceptive pill, blood pressure tablets, alendronic acid, and Ventolin.

Participants were asked if they had ever taken the Rorschach before. Only one participant indicated that she had been given the test previously when she was at university as part of a course she had completed in psychological assessment.

The administration of the Rorschach followed the standardized procedure as set out in the Comprehensive System workbook (fifth edition; Exner, 2001). Protocols with fewer than 14 responses were to be excluded from the study, as these protocols are considered to be invalid according to the Comprehensive System. No protocols had to be discarded for this reason. In addition to taking the Rorschach and filling out the demographics form, all participants completed the CORE-Short Form A (Core Outcomes in Routine Evaluation; see Barkham et al., 2010) in order to gather data on reported levels of distress in the sample for further analysis.

Examiners recorded the Rorschach responses in writing during each test administration. After each administration was completed, they typed up and scored the verbatim records. Each examiner received feedback on their scoring of their third protocol from a Rorschach expert from another European country in order to check on possible scoring issues at an early stage in the study. Once each examiner had completed all of their protocols, all of the records were then passed to a second examiner in the study who reviewed the scoring and communicated with the examiner who had administered that protocol about any suggested corrections. If the correction was accepted by the examiner, it was then entered into

Table 1. Results for gender

Gender	General population	Our sample	
		Number	Percentage
Male	49%	46	52%
Female	51%	42	48%
Total	100%	88	100%

the database. If the examiner disagreed with the correction, the scoring dilemma in question was then passed to a third examiner in the group of five examiners who then cast the deciding vote.

Rorschach data were entered into the computer program called CHESSSS (Code for Hermann: Enhanced Structural Summary and Supplementary Scales; see Fontan et al., 2013). All 88 protocols were then passed to the sixth author who did not participate in the data collection and who is from a different European country in order to ensure that the scoring within the group was calibrated by someone from a different setting and to correct for any possible local scoring bias. The sixth author's scoring was compared with the agreed scoring that the group had reached. Any differences were discussed with the first author. Some of the differences concerned a judgment call (such as whether to score for form quality unusual or form quality minus). In these cases, the original scoring was retained. Some differences were found to be due to a simple error (such as a missing score for a pair because of an oversight). In these cases, the error was corrected. Certain other scoring differences required more discussion before a consensus could be reached. Most of these concerned the special scores, for example, a response where the group of examiners from England scored for INCOM2 and the sixth author scored for INCOM1 and ALOG.

In order to calculate interscorer reliability, one quarter of the protocols (22 in total) were randomly selected and rescored by the seventh author who had not participated in data collection and who was blind to the scoring that had been assigned by the aforementioned process.

Results

Demographics

We attempted to match our sample with the 2011 Office for National Statistics census data on the variables of gender, ethnicity, age, marital status, level of education, occupation, and geographical region (Office for National Statistics, 2011). The results for gender, ethnicity, and age are given in Tables 1, 2, and 3 for each

Table 2. Results for ethnicity

Ethnicity	General population	Our sample	
		Number	Percentage
White	86%	80	91%
Asian	8%	2	2%
Black	3%	3	3%
Mixed	2%	2	2%
Other	1%	1	1%
Total	100%	88	99%

Note. Percentages have been rounded.

Table 3. Results for age

Age range	General population	Our sample	
		Number	Percentage
18–24	13%	14	16%
25–29	12%	8	9%
30–34	11%	12	14%
35–39	11%	5	6%
40–44	12%	15	17%
45–49	12%	11	12%
50–54	10%	10	11%
55–59	9%	7	8%
60–65	10%	6	7%
Total	100%	88	100%

variable. Percentages are rounded to the nearest whole number and thus may not equal 100.

Concerning marital status, we had the following groups in our study: single, cohabiting, civil partnership, married, separated, divorced, and widowed. It was not clear how the data in the census treated couples who were cohabiting. The category of civil partnerships consisted of only 0.2% of the population in the census data. Therefore, for the purposes of comparison, we collapsed cohabiting and civil partnerships into the married category. The category of cohabiting was endorsed by 14 of our participants. None of them endorsed the category of civil partnership. The results for marital status are given in Table 4.

No significant differences were found between the present sample and the general population for gender ($\chi^2 = 0.36$, $df = 1$, $p = .55$), ethnicity ($\chi^2 = 5.79$, $df = 4$,

Table 4. Results for marital status

Marital status	General population	Our sample	
		Number	Percentage
Single	34%	35	40%
Married, civil, cohab	47%	44	46%
Separated	3%	4	4%
Divorced	9%	9	10%
Widowed	7%	None	0%
Total	100%	88	100%

Note. Civil = civil partnership; cohab. = cohabiting.

$p = .22$), age ($\chi^2 = 7.73$, $df = 8$, $p = .46$), and marital status ($\chi^2 = 8.525$, $df = 4$, $p = .07$).

For education, the six categories that were derived from the census data are: (1) Level 0: no academic, vocational, or professional qualifications; (2) Level 1: one or more O levels, CSEs, GCSEs, or O grades (each at any grade), Intermediate 1 and 2, NVQ Level 1, Foundation GNVQ; (3) Level 2: five or more O levels, CSEs (Grade1), GCSEs (Grade A–C) or O grades, one A level, one or more AS levels, Higher Grades, NVQ Level 2, Intermediate GNVQ or equivalents; (4) Level 3: two or more A levels, four or more AS levels, Higher Grades, Higher School Certificate, NVQ Level 3, Advanced GNVQ or equivalents; (5) Level 4: First Degree, Higher Degree, NVQ Levels 4–5, HNC, HND, Qualified Teacher Status, Qualified Medical Doctor, Dentist, Nurse, Midwife, Health Visitor or equivalents; (6) Level 5: other qualifications (e.g. City and Guilds, RSA/OCR, BTEC, Edexcel)/level unknown. Table 5 shows the results for this variable.

The educational levels that we used come from the census in this country and reflect the examination and qualification system in this country. In order to assist with comparisons with other countries, we calculated the average number of years of education in our sample using estimates for number of years corresponding to the different levels listed earlier. This yielded an average of 13.64 years with a standard deviation of 1.55 years and a range of 10–18 years.

For occupation, participants were asked what work they did and their responses were divided into the following six categories as derived from the census data: (1) A: higher managerial, administrative, or professional; (2) B: intermediate managerial, administrative, or professional; (3) C1: supervisory or clerical, junior managerial, administrative, or professional; (4) C2: skilled manual workers; (5) D: semi- and unskilled workers; (6) unemployed.

We included participants who were in full-time education (two participants), who had taken early retirement (one participant), and who were on long-term

Table 5. Results for education

Level of education	General population	Our sample	
		Number	Percentage
0	8%	1	1%
1	12%	6	7%
2	17%	15	17%
3	17%	17	19%
4	34%	46	52%
5	12%	3	3%
Total	100%	88	99%

Note. Percentages have been rounded. See text for explanation of educational levels.

Table 6. Results for occupation

Occupational level	General population	Our sample	
		Number	Percentage
A and B	39%	39	44%
C1 and C2	38%	33	38%
D	17%	6	7%
Unemployed	6%	10	11%
Total	100%	88	100%

Note. See text for explanation of occupational levels.

sickness benefit (one participant) in this last category for the unemployed. We amalgamated A and B into one category and C1 and C2 into another category, leaving us with four categories for occupation. Table 6 shows the results for this variable.

For location, we broke down England into nine regions: North East, North West, Yorkshire, East Midlands, West Midlands, East, London, South East, and South West. Table 7 shows the results for this variable.

Significant differences were found for the demographic variables of education (χ^2 = 25.811, df = 5, p < .0001), occupation (χ^2 = 10.69, df = 3, p < .02), and location (χ^2 = 44.86, df = 8, p < .0001). In particular, for education the present sample includes more participants with a Level 4 qualification and not enough in Level 0. This may be because more highly educated people are more likely to volunteer to participate in research and also because researchers are more likely to know and have contacts among groups of highly educated people. For occupation, the sample includes too many participants in the unemployed category (who have time to participate in a research study) and not enough semi- and unskilled workers

Table 7. Results for location

Region	General population	Our sample	
		Number	Percentage
North East	5%	2	2%
North West	13%	15	17%
Yorkshire	10%	3	3%
East Midlands	9%	None	0%
West Midlands	11%	1	1%
East	11%	14	16%
London	15%	19	21%
South East	16%	26	30%
South West	10%	8	9%
Total	100%	88	99%

Note. Percentages have been rounded.

Table 8. Results for interscorer reliability

Variables	κ	Interpretation
Location	0.96	Excellent
DQ	0.96	Excellent
Determinants	0.88	Excellent
FQ	0.75	Excellent
Pair	0.96	Excellent
Contents	0.92	Excellent
Popular	0.97	Excellent
Zf	0.92	Excellent
Sum6	0.58	Fair
Other special scores[a]	0.90	Excellent
All special scores	0.84	Excellent

Note. $N = 22$. [a]This includes all the special scores apart from DV, DR, INCOM, FABCOM, ALOG, and CONTAM.

(who may be less available). For location, there are too many participants in the South East and not enough in Yorkshire and the Midlands. This is a function of where the examiners were based.

The CORE Data

The mean score for the CORE short form A in our sample was 6.7 with a standard deviation of 5. Connell et al. (2007) obtained a mean CORE score of 4.8, with a standard deviation of 4.3, for 553 adults in the general population. Comparing our result with their results, the effect size of the difference between our sample and theirs is Cohen's $d = 0.41$, which is a small effect size. Connell et al. (2007) also reported on results for the CORE for a clinical sample of 10,761 patients, with a mean of 18.3 and a standard deviation of 7.1. The effect size of the difference between our sample and this clinical sample is Cohen's $d = 1.88$, which is very large. According to these comparisons, it would appear that our sample is slightly more distressed on average than the general population but far less distressed than the clinical population.

A cut-off for identifying a clinically significant level of distress has been given as a score of greater than 10 by Connell et al. (2007). In our sample, the minimum score obtained on the CORE was 0 and the maximum was 22.78, with 18 participants scoring above the cut-off of 10. It would therefore appear that 20% of our participants were experiencing a clinically significant level of distress at the time when they took the Rorschach.

The Rorschach Data

The results for the 22 randomly selected protocols that were rescored to investigate interscorer reliability were analyzed and kappa coefficients were calculated between the two sets of scores, as shown in Table 8.

Results for the statistical properties for the Rorschach variables for our sample are presented in Table A1 in the Appendix.

The values for Lambda are based on 87 participants because one participant gave only pure form responses and therefore Lambda cannot be computed in this case. Although it could be argued that this protocol was not valid, we decided to retain it as the number of responses was 21 and there was no other reason for it to be excluded. We note that Ritzler and Exner (1995) advise researchers not to exclude high Lambda protocols in studies where one is attempting to obtain a representative sample.

We give the comparisons between our sample and Exner's (2007) sample in Table A2 in the Appendix. We obtained large differences for eight variables, moderate differences for 28 variables, small differences for 43 variables, and no significant differences for 34 variables. Large differences are defined as effect sizes between 0.80 and 1.29, medium differences are between 0.50 and 0.79, and small differences are between 0.20 and 0.49 (Ellis, 2009). The eight variables for which large differences were obtained are FQxo, CF, SumColor, XA%, WDA%, X+%, X−%, and PER.

We give the comparisons between our sample and the international reference sample (Meyer et al., 2007) in Table A3 in the Appendix. There were no large differences for any of the variables and a moderate difference on one variable only (Ay), with the English sample obtaining a higher mean.

For clinical interpretation, it is useful to have frequency data for the indices. Accordingly, we present these figures in Tables 9–17 for S-Con, PTI, DEPI, CDI, HVI, EB style, Form quality deviations, *D* and Adjusted *D*. For OBS, none of our sample obtained a positive result.

Table 9. Frequency data for S-CON

S-CON value	N
1	2
2	15
3	10
4	21
5	11
6	21
7	4
8	3
10	1
Total	88

Table 10. Frequency data for PTI

PTI value	N
0	51
1	16
2	12
3	8
5	1
Total	88

Table 11. Frequency data for DEPI

DEPI value	N
1	2
2	24
3	17
4	16
5	15
6	13
7	1
Total	88

Table 12. Frequency data for CDI

CDI value	N
0	1
1	15
2	26
3	22
4	21
5	3
Total	88

Table 13. Frequency data for HVI

HVI value	N
Negative	76
Positive	12
Total	88

Table 14. Frequency data for EB

EB	N
Ambitent	28
EB < 4	19
Introversive	25
Extratensive	16
Total	88

Table 15. Frequency data for *D*

D value	N
−8	1
−6	1
−3	1
−2	11
−1	17
0	41
1	12
2	4
Total	88

Table 16. Frequency data for Adjusted *D*

Adj D value	N
−4	1
−3	1
−2	4
−1	14
0	42
1	17
2	8
4	1
Total	88

Table 17. Frequency data for form quality deviations

Form quality	Percentage
XA% > 0.89	18%
XA% < 0.70	26%
WDA% < 0.85	64%
WDA% < 0.75	25%
X+% < 0.55	57%
Xu% > 0.20	60%
X−% > 0.20	45%
X−% > 0.30	14%

Discussion

Firstly, and most importantly, the number of responses was not significantly different for our sample as compared with either the Exner (2007) sample or the international reference sample (Meyer et al., 2007). This supports the conclusion that our administration did not deviate significantly from the standardized procedure, at least with regard to examinees' ability to generate responses to the inkblots. It is also very important to have confirmed excellent interscorer reliability, with a somewhat lower value for Sum6. We consider that Sum6 might be lower because the protocols were rescored by a native French speaker and it is very hard for a nonnative speaker to score accurately for deviant verbalizations in particular.

Large differences were found for several variables relating to form quality when comparing our sample with Exner's sample. For example, only 18% of our sample had XA% > 0.89 compared with 45% of Exner's sample. Conversely, 45% of our sample had X−% > 0.20, whereas only 10% of his sample did. In general, our sample gave fewer good form quality responses and more form quality minus responses. However, it is also worth noting that our sample did not differ significantly on any of the form quality variables as compared with the international reference sample. As Silva and Pires (2011) observed, lower form quality is often found in normative studies outside the United States, suggesting that there may be a benefit to each country drawing up its own form quality table.

The finding of many more differences between our sample and Exner's (2007) sample as compared with the number of differences with the international reference sample is not surprising given that the international reference sample contains an amalgamation of data sets from 17 countries whereas Exner's sample is from the United States only. For the 143 variables listed in both studies, the standard deviations are lower for Exner's sample in all but 18 variables, reflecting the likelihood that the international reference sample is much more diverse than his sample. Lower standard deviations make it more likely that one will find significant differences.

As compared with Exner's (2007) US sample, we found large differences on two variables relating to use of color (CF and SumColor), while smaller but still significant differences were found for FC and for the Affective Ratio. One of our participants turned out to be color blind. Corsino (1985) found that color blind individuals gave fewer pure C responses and Hayslip, McBride, Lowman, and Aronson (1992) found that in older adults, color blind individuals appeared affectively constricted as compared with their peers who were not color blind. However, in our case, the color-blind participant was extratensive and obtained an Affective ratio of 0.86, and FC: CF +C was 0:8, with one pure color response; therefore, this particular protocol did not contribute to the differences in the use of color across the two samples.

Cross-cultural differences in emotional arousal level have consistently been found (Lim, 2016), with the higher levels of emotional expression in the individualistic cultures of the West commonly attributed to the need to influence others (Tsai, Miao, Seppala, Fung, & Yeung, 2007). While there has been very little research exploring trans-Atlantic differences, a 2012 poll by Gallup that measured positive and negative emotions in 150 countries found that residents of the United States scored higher than those in the UK on an overall ranking of emotionality, a finding reflected in American literature, which since 1960 has had increasingly more emotional mood content than its British counterpart (Acerbi, Lampos, Garnett, & Bentley, 2013; Clifton, 2012). We therefore suggest that our Rorschach findings are consistent with the hypothesis that the English are on average somewhat less emotionally expressive than the Americans.

Thirdly, a large difference was found for the special score, PER. Our English sample gave fewer PER as compared with Exner's sample or with the international reference sample. We speculate that the English tend to be somewhat self-effacing and to hesitate to refer to themselves as compared with Americans.

Our sample would appear to be in more distress than the Exner sample, as judging by our findings of 11% with a PTI of 3 or more compared with less than 1% in Exner's sample, 33% with a DEPI of 5 or more compared with 14% in Exner's sample, and 30% with an Adjusted D of less than 0 compared with 13% of Exner's sample. As Rosso, Camoirano, and Schiaffino (2015) point out, nonpatient samples are not necessarily psychologically healthy and 20% of our sample reported clinically significant distress; we aim to investigate this further to see whether there are any relationships between our Rorschach variables and the CORE results.

The data for Exner's (2007) sample were gathered between 1999 and 2005, whereas our data were gathered between 2014 and 2016. One hypothesis is that our sample appears to be more distressed on the Rorschach as compared with Exner's (2007) sample owing to a real difference in the level of distress in the general population over time. We know that anxiety and depression are markedly higher than they were in earlier eras; this is true in the United States (Cohen & Janicki-Deverts, 2012) and in the UK, where depression and anxiety levels are rising at the same time as overall satisfaction with health (including mental health) is declining. Indeed, data from the Office for National Statistics show that mixed anxiety and depression is the most common mental disorder in Britain, with 7.8% of people meeting the diagnostic criteria (National Institute for Clinical Excellence, 2011). We also note that poverty increases the risk of mental health problems (Fell & Hewstone, 2015) and unemployment is a risk factor for depression (Montgomery, Cook, Bartley, & Wadsworth, 1999), thus having too many participants in the unemployed category may have contributed to an elevated level of distress in our sample.

Limitations

The main limitation of this study is the small sample size; it is representative of the general population on gender, ethnicity, age, and marital status but there are significant differences on the demographic variables of location, education, and occupation. Concerning location, although the relative lack of participants in the Midlands and Yorkshire is regrettable, we doubt that this has had a significant impact on the Rorschach variables.

However, number of years in education has been associated with Rorschach variables that relate to complexity and cognitive synthesis (Meyer, Giromini, Viglione, Reese, & Mihura, 2015). We have not yet investigated the question of any relationships between the demographic variables and the Rorschach in our sample but our finding of a moderate effect size for Ay in our sample as compared with the international reference sample (Meyer et al., 2007) suggests that the English might intellectualize a bit more than the average *international composite* person because Ay is a component in the intellectualization index. Looking at the comparison for this index itself, there was a small effect size with our sample obtaining a mean of 2.98 as compared with the mean of 2.35 for the international reference sample. We note that Mazzorana Ribeiro, Semer, and Yazigi (2011), in their normative study of Brazilian children from public and private schools, obtained a significant difference for the intellectualization index in favor of children in private schools, suggesting that there may be a relationship between education and this index. It is therefore possible that the bias toward more well-educated participants in our sample as compared with census data has contributed to this finding for Ay.

Conclusion

We look forward to carrying out further analysis of our results looking at any relationships between the CORE results and Rorschach variables. For now, we would recommend that clinicians using the Rorschach in England refer to our data in addition to other published normative data in order to arrive at the most accurate conclusions concerning their patients. In particular, we would hesitate to make statements about difficulties with perceptual accuracy unless an English examinee's results indicated that this was markedly lower when using the average values for XA%, WDA%, X+%, and X−% that were obtained in our sample as a benchmark.

Acknowledgments

With special thanks to Dr. Vera Campo for her assistance with scoring and to Dr. Concepcion Sendin for the Spanish translation.

References

Acerbi, A., Lampos, V., Garnett, P., & Bentley, A. (2013). The expression of emotions in 20th century books. *PLoS One, 8*(3), e59030. https://doi.org/10.1371/journal.pone.0059030

Barkham, M., Mellor-Clark, J., Connell, J., Evans, C., Evans, R., & Margison, F. (2010). Clinical Outcomes in Routine Evaluation (CORE) – the CORE measures and system: Measuring, monitoring and managing quality evaluation in the psychological therapies. In M. Barkham, G. E. Hardy, & J. Mellor-Clark (Eds.), *Developing and delivering practice-based evidence: A guide for the psychological therapies* (pp. 175–219). Chichester, UK: Wiley-Blackwell.

Clifton, J. (2012). *Singapore ranks as least emotional country in the world*. Retrieved from http://www.gallup.com/poll/158882/singapore-ranks-least-emotional-country-world.aspx

Cohen, S., & Janicki-Deverts, D. (2012). Who's stressed? Distributions of psychological stress in the United States in probability samples from 1983, 2006, and 2009. *Journal of Applied Social Psychology, 42*, 1320–1334. https://doi.org/10.1111/j.1559-1816.2012.00900.x

Connell, J., Barkham, M., Stiles, W. B., Twigg, E., Singleton, N., Evans, O., & Miles, J. N. V. (2007). Distribution of CORE-OM scores in a general population, clinical cut-off points and comparison with the CIS-R. *British Journal of Psychiatry, 190*, 69–74. https://doi.org/10.1192/bjp.bp.105.017657

Corsino, B. V. (1985). Color blindness and Rorschach color responsivity. *Journal of Personality Assessment, 49*, 533–534.

Ellis, P. D. (2009). *Thresholds for interpreting effect sizes*. Retrieved from http://www.polyu.edu.hk/mm/effectsizefaqs/thresholds_for_interpreting_effect_sizes2.html

Exner, J. E. (2001). *A Rorschach workbook for the comprehensive system:* (5th ed.). Asheville, NC: Rorschach Workshops.

Exner, J. E. (2003). *The Rorschach: A comprehensive system. Volume 1: Basic foundations and principles of interpretation*. New York, NY: Wiley.

Exner, J. E. (2007). A new US adult nonpatient sample. *Journal of Personality Assessment, 89*(S1), S154–S158. https://doi.org/10.1080/00223890701583523

Fell, B., & Hewstone, M. (2015). *Psychological perspectives on poverty*. York, UK: Joseph Rowntree Foundation Retrieved from https://www.jrf.org.uk/report/psychological-perspectives-poverty

Fontan, P., Andronikof, A., Nicodemo, D., Al Nyssani, L., Guilheri, J., Hansen, K. G., ..., & Nakamura, N. (2013). CHESSSS: A free software solution to score and compute the Rorschach Comprehensive System and Supplementary Scales. *Rorschachiana, 34*, 56–82. https://doi.org/10.1027/1192-5604/a000040

Hayslip, B., McBride, P. A., Lowman, R. L., & Aronson, H. J. (1992). Color vision deficits and Rorschach performance in aged persons. *The International Journal of Aging & Human Development, 34*, 165–173. https://doi.org/10.2190/3VP2-X2J1-KQT2-DUV1

Lim, N. (2016). Cultural differences in emotion: Differences in emotional arousal level between the East and the West. *Integrative Medicine Research, 5*, 105–109. https://doi.org/10.1016/j.imr.2016.03.004

Mazzorana Ribeiro, R. K. S., Semer, N. L., & Yazigi, L. (2011). Rorschach Comprehensive System norms in Brazilian children from public and private schools. *Psicologia: Reflexão e Crítica, 24*, 671–684. https://doi.org/10.1590/S0102-79722011000400007

Meyer, G. J., Erdberg, P., & Shaffer, T. W. (2007). Toward international normative reference data for the comprehensive system. *Journal of Personality Assessment, 89*(S1), S201–S216. https://doi.org/10.1080/00223890701629342

Meyer, G. J., Giromini, L., Viglione, D. J., Reese, J. B., & Mihura, J. L. (2015). The association of gender, ethnicity, age, and education with Rorschach scores. *Assessment, 22*, 46–64. https://doi.org/10.1177/1073191114544358

Montgomery, S. M., Cook, D. G., Bartley, M. J., & Wadsworth, M. E. J. (1999). Unemployment pre-dates symptoms of depression and anxiety resulting in medical consultations in young men. *International Journal of Epidemiology, 28*, 95–100. https://doi.org/10.1093/ije/28.1.95

National Institute for Clinical Excellence. (2011). *Common mental health disorders: guidance and guidelines.* Retrieved from http://www.nice.org.uk/guidance/cg123

Office for National Statistics (2011). *2011 census.* Retrieved from https://www.ons.gov.uk/census/2011census

Ritzler, B. A., & Exner, J. E. (1995). Special issues in subject selection and design. In John E. Exner (Ed.), *Issues and methods in Rorschach research* (pp. 123–143). New York, NY: Routledge.

Rosso, A. M., Camoirano, A., & Schiaffino, G. (2015). Are individuals in Rorschach nonpatient samples truly psychologically healthy? Data of a sample of 212 adult nonpatients from Italy. *Rorschachiana, 36*, 112–155. https://doi.org/10.1027/1192-5604/a000052

Silva, D. R., & Pires, A. A. (2011). One more datum on Rorschach form quality. *Journal of Personality Assessment, 93*, 316–322. https://doi.org/10.1080/00223891.2011.558877

Tsai, J. L., Miao, F. F., Seppala, E., Fung, H. H., & Yeung, D. Y. (2007). Influence and adjustment goals: Sources of cultural differences in ideal affect. *Journal of Personality and Social Psychology, 92*, 1102–1117. https://doi.org/10.1037/0022-3514.92.6.1102

Received December 12, 2017
Revision received March 3, 2018
Accepted April 20, 2018
Published online November 9, 2018

Kari Carstairs
7 Mayfield Road
Bromley
Kent
BR1 2HB
UK
kari@carstairspsych.co.uk

Appendix

Table A1. Statistics for Rorschach variables

N = 88	M	SD	Min	Max	Frequency	Mdn	Mode	Skewness	Kurtosis
R	22.82	6.97	14	50	88	21	20	1.49	2.51
W	8.72	4.54	1	27	88	8	7	1.2	2.48
D	11.07	4.7	2	23	88	11	10	0.3	−0.23
Dd	3.03	2.93	0	13	69	2	0	1.15	1.05
S	2.82	2.11	0	9	78	2.5	1	0.72	−0.05
DQ+	6.02	3.84	0	21	86	6	7	1.1	2.12
DQo	15.92	5.8	4	34	88	15	18	0.85	0.92
DQv	0.74	1.2	0	6	33	0	0	2.04	4.89
DQv/+	0.14	0.38	0	2	11	0	0	2.79	7.66
FQx+	0.3	0.7	0	3	16	0	0	2.43	5.23
FQxo	11.57	4.18	4	24	88	11	12	0.64	0.41
FQxu	5.74	3.53	0	18	87	5	3	1.28	2.08
FQx−	4.5	2.88	0	14	84	4	4	0.98	1.55
FQxnone	0.67	1.16	0	6	30	0	0	2.12	5.09
MQ+	0.15	0.42	0	2	11	0	0	2.94	8.51
MQo	2.49	1.73	0	8	80	2	3	1	1.19
MQu	0.55	0.82	0	4	34	0	0	1.67	3.16
MQ−	0.74	0.99	0	5	40	0	0	1.5	2.84
MQnone	0.08	0.38	0	2	4	0	0	4.78	21.89
S−	1	1.01	0	4	54	1	0	0.76	−0.17
M	4	2.63	0	16	85	3	3	1.49	4.19
FM	3.01	1.89	0	12	81	3	3	1.12	4.51
m	1.66	1.86	0	10	63	1	1	1.99	5.14
FM + m	4.67	2.75	0	13	82	4.5	5	0.45	0.2
FC	1.92	1.66	0	6	66	2	0	0.68	-0.2
CF	1.45	1.65	0	7	57	1	0	1.51	2.27
C	0.49	0.8	0	3	29	0	0	1.61	1.82
Cn	0	0	0	0	0	0	0	N/A	N/A
Sum Color	3.86	2.55	0	12	81	3	3	0.79	0.71
WsumC	3.15	2.39	0	11.5	81	2.5	2	1.14	1.37
SumC'	1.44	1.52	0	5	60	1	0	1.12	0.36
SumT	0.52	0.88	0	4	31	0	0	2.13	4.91
SumV	0.52	0.93	0	5	30	0	0	2.48	7.44
SumY	1.41	1.59	0	7	51	1	0	1.13	0.89

(Continued on next page)

Table A1. (Continued)

N = 88	M	SD	Min	Max	Frequency	Mdn	Mode	Skewness	Kurtosis
Sum Shading	3.9	3.24	0	19	80	3	2	1.64	4.56
Fr + rF	0.39	0.7	0	3	25	0	0	1.95	3.55
FD	0.68	0.94	0	4	42	0	0	1.87	3.9
F	9.69	5.12	1	31	88	9	5	1.34	3.26
(2)	6.61	3.28	1	16	88	6	6	0.48	0.02
3r + (2)/R	0.35	0.14	0.04	0.79	88	0.35	0.25	0.05	0.29
Lambda	0.92	0.85	0.06	4.67	87	0.71	1	2.56	7.66
F%	0.42	0.18	0.05	1	88	0.42	0.5	0.62	0.53
EA	7.15	3.59	0	17.5	87	6.5	6	0.59	0.38
es	8.57	5.14	0	28	86	7.5	7	1.06	1.83
D score	−0.41	1.45	−8	2	16	0	0	−2.25	9.65
AdjD	0.09	1.17	−4	4	26	0	0	−0.18	2.26
a (active)	4.7	2.98	0	18	85	4	4	1.44	4.22
p (passive)	4.05	2.33	0	10	84	3	3	0.47	−0.39
Ma	2.06	1.81	0	9	75	1.5	1	1.31	1.78
Mp	1.93	1.47	0	7	69	2	2	0.5	0.3
Intellect	2.98	2.59	0	12	74	3	3	1.26	1.83
Zf	12.84	5.65	1	30	88	12	10	1.09	1.83
Zd	−0.48	4.8	−15.5	7.5	37	−0.5	−0.5	−0.38	−0.02
Blends	3.75	3.12	0	15	76	3	2	1.09	1.25
Blends/R	0.17	0.14	0	0.79	76	0.14	0	1.32	3.61
Col-Shd Blends	0.52	0.9	0	4	29	0	0	1.89	3.19
Afr	0.55	0.16	0.16	1.2	88	0.54	0.5	1.01	2.8
PC%	0.35	0.07	0.14	0.55	88	0.35	0.33	−0.02	1.37
Populars	5.22	2.02	1	10	88	5	5	0.23	−0.46
XA%	0.78	0.12	0.43	1	88	0.78	0.67	−0.23	−0.12
WDA%	0.8	0.11	0.53	1	88	0.8	0.75	−0.37	−0.28
X+%	0.53	0.16	0.2	0.9	88	0.51	0.5	0.39	−0.43
X−%	0.19	0.11	0	0.57	84	0.2	0	0.53	0.79
Xu%	0.25	0.12	0	0.55	87	0.23	0.25	0.42	−0.42
Isolate/R	0.18	0.13	0	0.53	85	0.16	0.25	0.89	0.27
H	2.45	2.21	0	15	80	2	1	2.67	11.45
(H)	0.92	0.96	0	3	51	1	0	0.72	−0.53
Hd	1.76	1.54	0	7	70	1	1	0.94	0.47
(Hd)	0.85	0.95	0	5	51	1	0	1.44	3.18
Hx	0.34	0.83	0	5	18	0	0	3.25	12.67

(Continued on next page)

Table A1. (Continued)

N = 88	M	SD	Min	Max	Frequency	Mdn	Mode	Skewness	Kurtosis
All H Cont	5.99	3.19	1	19	88	5	4	1.52	3.59
A	8.09	3.16	3	19	88	8	8	1.12	1.81
(A)	0.31	0.57	0	3	23	0	0	2.11	5.29
Ad	2.75	1.82	0	7	79	3	3	0.39	−0.43
(Ad)	0.17	0.41	0	2	14	0	0	2.29	4.68
An	1.28	1.21	0	5	61	1	1	0.9	0.32
Art	1.26	1.47	0	7	55	1	0	1.82	4.55
Ay	1.17	1.26	0	5	53	1	0	0.97	0.24
Bl	0.27	0.58	0	2	18	0	0	2.04	3.03
Bt	1.31	1.2	0	5	62	1	1	0.82	0.2
Cg	1.68	1.97	0	10	59	1	0	1.88	4.6
Cl	0.13	0.4	0	2	9	0	0	3.36	11.38
Ex	0.16	0.52	0	3	9	0	0	3.65	13.74
Fi	0.31	0.72	0	3	18	0	0	2.72	7.26
Food	0.3	0.53	0	2	23	0	0	1.61	1.74
Ge	0.34	0.66	0	3	23	0	0	2.22	5.19
Hh	1.23	1.4	0	8	58	1	1	2.08	6.52
Ls	0.95	1.2	0	6	47	1	0	1.59	3.04
Na	0.74	1.29	0	7	35	0	0	2.64	8.42
Sc	1.67	1.66	0	7	65	1	1	1.49	2.51
Sx	0.59	0.97	0	5	33	0	0	2.08	4.98
Xy	0.15	0.42	0	2	11	0	0	2.94	8.51
Idio	0.49	0.66	0	2	35	0	0	1.02	−0.1
DV	0.55	1.06	0	6	28	0	0	2.9	10.42
INCOM	0.92	0.91	0	3	54	1	0	0.72	−0.32
DR	0.38	0.72	0	4	25	0	0	2.57	8.38
FABCOM	0.45	0.69	0	3	31	0	0	1.44	1.5
DV2	0	0	0	0	0	0	0	N/A	N/A
INC2	0.2	0.53	0	2	13	0	0	2.57	5.61
DR2	0.01	0.11	0	1	1	0	0	9.38	88
FAB2	0.24	0.57	0	3	17	0	0	3.08	11.36
ALOG	0.28	0.71	0	3	16	0	0	2.87	8
CONTAM	0.01	0.11	0	1	1	0	0	9.38	88
Sum 6 SpSc	3.05	2.64	0	15	75	2.5	1	1.46	3.83
Lvl 2 SpSc	0.45	0.79	0	4	29	0	0	2.18	5.56
Wsum6	9.39	9.4	0	59	75	7	0	2.14	8.04

(Continued on next page)

Table A1. (Continued)

N = 88	M	SD	Min	Max	Frequency	Mdn	Mode	Skewness	Kurtosis
AB	0.27	0.69	0	4	15	0	0	3.01	10.4
AG	0.74	0.96	0	5	42	0	0	1.57	3.36
COP	1.28	1.23	0	5	61	1	1	0.99	0.65
CP	0.01	0.11	0	1	1	0	0	9.38	88
GHR	3.53	2.2	0	12	84	3.5	2	0.89	1.65
PHR	3.2	2.48	0	11	80	3	4	1.03	0.88
MOR	1	1.16	0	4	49	1	0	1.07	0.25
PER	0.25	0.61	0	3	16	0	0	2.9	9
PSV	0.24	0.48	0	2	19	0	0	1.87	2.77

Note. N/A not applicable.

Table A2. Comparisons with Exner's sample

Variable	CS		England		England vs. CS	
	M	SD	M	SD	Cohen's d	Effect size
R	23.36	5.68	22.82	6.97	−0.08	
W	9.1	3.7	8.72	4.54	−0.09	
D	12.66	4.75	11.07	4.7	−0.34	*
Dd	1.6	2.06	3.03	2.93	0.56	**
S	2.37	1.97	2.82	2.11	0.22	*
DQ+	8.43	3.07	6.02	3.84	−0.69	**
DQo	14.29	4.66	15.92	5.8	0.31	*
DQv	0.37	0.72	0.74	1.2	0.37	*
DQv/+	0.27	0.61	0.14	0.38	−0.26	*
FQx+	0.54	0.93	0.3	0.7	−0.29	*
FQxo	15.09	3.22	11.57	4.18	−0.94	***
FQxu	4.85	2.93	5.74	3.53	0.27	*
FQx−	2.73	2.01	4.5	2.88	0.71	**
FQxNone	0.15	0.41	0.67	1.16	0.6	**
MQ+	0.42	0.72	0.15	0.42	−0.46	*
MQo	3.74	1.79	2.49	1.73	−0.71	**
MQu	0.44	0.81	0.55	0.82	0.13	
MQ−	0.23	0.57	0.74	0.99	0.63	**
MQNone	0.01	0.08	0.08	0.38	0.25	*
S−	0.58	0.89	1	1.01	0.44	*
M	4.83	2.18	4	2.63	−0.34	*
FM	4.04	1.9	3.01	1.89	−0.54	**
m	1.57	1.34	1.66	1.86	0.06	
FC	2.97	1.78	1.92	1.66	−0.61	**
CF	2.8	1.64	1.45	1.65	−0.82	***
C	0.17	0.45	0.49	0.8	0.49	*
Cn	0	0.07	0	0	0	
SumColor	5.95	2.47	3.86	2.55	−0.83	***
WSumC	4.54	1.98	3.15	2.39	−0.63	**
Sum C'	1.6	1.35	1.44	1.52	−0.11	
Sum T	1.01	0.69	0.52	0.88	−0.62	**
Sum V	0.35	0.77	0.52	0.93	0.2	*
Sum Y	0.97	1.2	1.41	1.59	0.31	*
SumShading	3.94	2.45	3.9	3.24	−0.01	
Fr + rF	0.2	0.67	0.39	0.7	0.28	*

(Continued on next page)

Table A2. (Continued)

	CS		England		England vs. CS	
Variable	M	SD	M	SD	Cohen's d	Effect size
FD	1.43	1.15	0.68	0.94	−0.71	**
F	7.91	3.7	9.69	5.12	0.4	*
Pair	8.82	3.08	6.61	3.28	−0.69	**
3r + (2)/R	0.4	0.3	0.35	0.14	−0.21	*
Lambda	0.58	0.37	0.92	0.85	0.52	**
PureF%	0.34	0.13	0.42	0.18	0.51	**
FM + m	5.61	2.51	4.67	2.75	−0.36	*
EA	9.37	3	7.15	3.59	−0.67	**
es	9.55	4.01	8.57	5.14	−0.21	*
D score	−0.12	0.99	−0.41	1.45	−0.23	*
AdjD	0.19	0.83	0.09	1.17	−0.1	
a (active)	6.76	2.87	4.7	2.98	−0.7	**
p (passive)	3.73	2.34	4.05	2.33	0.14	
Ma	2.93	1.67	2.06	1.81	−0.5	**
Mp	1.93	1.37	1.93	1.47	0	
Intellect	2.17	2.15	2.98	2.59	0.34	*
Zf	13.45	4.22	12.84	5.65	−0.12	
Zd	0.25	3.71	−0.48	4.8	−0.17	
Blends	5.56	2.55	3.75	3.12	−0.64	**
Blends/R	0.24	0.1	0.17	0.14	−0.58	**
Col-ShdBld	0.67	0.93	0.52	0.9	−0.16	
Afr	0.61	0.17	0.55	0.16	−0.36	*
Populars	6.28	1.53	5.22	2.02	−0.59	**
XA%	0.88	0.07	0.78	0.12	−1.02	***
WDA%	0.91	0.06	0.8	0.11	−1.24	***
X+%	0.68	0.11	0.53	0.16	−1.09	***
X−%	0.11	0.07	0.19	0.11	0.87	***
Xu%	0.2	0.09	0.25	0.12	0.47	*
Isolate/R	0.19	0.09	0.18	0.13	−0.09	
H	3.18	1.7	2.45	2.21	−0.37	*
(H)	1.35	1.12	0.92	0.96	−0.41	*
Hd	1.14	1.26	1.76	1.54	0.44	*
(Hd)	0.62	0.87	0.85	0.95	0.25	*
Hx	0.15	0.5	0.34	0.83	0.28	*

(Continued on next page)

Table A2. (Continued)

	CS		England		England vs. CS	
Variable	M	SD	M	SD	Cohen's d	Effect size
H + (H) + Hd + (Hd)	6.29	2.66	5.99	3.19	−0.1	
A	8.18	2.56	8.09	3.16	−0.03	
(A)	0.42	0.69	0.31	0.57	−0.17	
Ad	2.9	1.65	2.75	1.82	−0.09	
(Ad)	0.13	0.38	0.17	0.41	0.1	
An	0.88	1.05	1.28	1.21	0.35	*
Art	1.19	1.42	1.26	1.47	0.05	
Ay	0.56	0.69	1.17	1.26	0.6	**
Bl	0.24	0.51	0.27	0.58	0.05	
Bt	2.22	1.52	1.31	1.2	−0.66	**
Cg	2.16	1.57	1.68	1.97	−0.27	*
Cl	0.16	0.41	0.13	0.4	−0.07	
Ex	0.21	0.47	0.16	0.52	−0.1	
Fi	0.81	0.84	0.31	0.72	−0.64	**
Food	0.26	0.55	0.3	0.53	0.07	
Ge	0.14	0.45	0.34	0.66	0.35	*
Hh	1.24	1.06	1.23	1.4	−0.01	
Ls	0.93	1.04	0.95	1.2	0.02	
Na	0.45	0.81	0.74	1.29	0.27	*
Sc	1.64	1.41	1.67	1.66	0.02	
Sx	0.19	0.53	0.59	0.97	0.51	**
Xy	0.08	0.28	0.15	0.42	0.2	*
Idiographic	0.34	0.65	0.49	0.66	0.23	*
DV	0.34	0.67	0.55	1.06	0.24	*
INCOM	0.71	0.93	0.92	0.91	0.23	*
DR	0.85	1.01	0.38	0.72	−0.54	**
FABCOM	0.45	0.77	0.45	0.69	0	
DV2	0	0.07	0	0	0	
INC2	0.06	0.25	0.2	0.53	0.34	*
DR2	0.03	0.18	0.01	0.11	−0.13	
FAB2	0.05	0.24	0.24	0.57	0.43	*
ALOG	0.04	0.21	0.28	0.71	0.46	*
CONTAM	0	0	0.01	0.11	0.13	
Sum 6 SpSc	2.54	1.9	3.05	2.64	0.22	*

(Continued on next page)

Table A2. (Continued)

	CS		England		England vs. CS	
Variable	M	SD	M	SD	Cohen's d	Effect size
Lvl 2 SpSc	0.15	0.39	0.45	0.79	0.48	*
WSum6	7.12	5.74	9.39	9.4	0.29	*
AB	0.21	0.56	0.27	0.69	0.1	
AG	0.89	1.02	0.74	0.96	−0.15	
COP	2.07	1.3	1.28	1.23	−0.62	**
CP	0.01	0.11	0.01	0.11	0	
Good HR	5.06	2.09	3.53	2.2	−0.71	**
Poor HR	2.12	1.81	3.2	2.48	0.5	**
MOR	0.93	1.01	1	1.16	0.06	
PER	0.99	1.1	0.25	0.61	−0.83	***
PSV	0.12	0.38	0.24	0.48	0.28	*

Notes. CS = Comprehensive System. Effect size: *small (between 0.20 and 0.49), **medium (between 0.50 and 0.79), ***large (between 0.80 and 1.29).

Table A3. Comparisons with the international reference sample

	International		England		England vs. CIRV	
Variable	M	SD	M	SD	Cohen's d	Effect size
R	22.31	7.9	22.82	6.97	0.07	
W	9.08	4.54	8.72	4.54	−0.08	
D	9.89	5.81	11.07	4.7	0.22	*
Dd	3.33	3.37	3.03	2.93	−0.1	
S	2.49	2.15	2.82	2.11	0.15	
DQ+	6.24	3.54	6.02	3.84	−0.06	
DQo	14.68	6.74	15.92	5.8	0.2	*
DQv	1.09	1.5	0.74	1.2	−0.26	*
DQv/+	0.29	0.67	0.14	0.38	−0.28	*
FQx+	0.21	0.68	0.3	0.7	0.13	
FQxo	11.11	3.74	11.57	4.18	0.12	
FQxu	6.2	3.93	5.74	3.53	−0.12	
FQx−	4.43	3.23	4.5	2.88	0.02	
FQxNone	0.33	0.71	0.67	1.16	0.35	*
MQ+	0.12	0.43	0.15	0.42	0.07	
MQo	2.26	1.66	2.49	1.73	0.14	
MQu	0.69	0.99	0.55	0.82	−0.15	
MQ−	0.63	1.05	0.74	0.99	0.11	
MQNone	0.03	0.2	0.08	0.38	0.16	
S−	0.87	1.15	1	1.01	0.12	
M	3.73	2.66	4	2.63	0.1	
FM	3.37	2.18	3.01	1.89	−0.18	
m	1.5	1.54	1.66	1.86	0.09	
FC	1.91	1.7	1.92	1.66	0.01	
CF	1.65	1.55	1.45	1.65	−0.12	
C	0.34	0.66	0.49	0.8	0.2	*
Cn	0.02	0.14	0	0	−0.2	*
SumColor	3.91	2.53	3.86	2.55	−0.02	
WSumC	3.11	2.17	3.15	2.39	0.02	
Sum C'	1.75	1.71	1.44	1.52	−0.19	
Sum T	0.65	0.91	0.52	0.88	−0.15	
Sum V	0.52	0.92	0.52	0.93	0	
Sum Y	1.34	1.63	1.41	1.59	0.04	
SumShading	4.29	3.48	3.9	3.24	−0.12	
Fr + rF	0.41	0.88	0.39	0.7	−0.03	

(Continued on next page)

Table A3. (Continued)

	International		England		England vs. CIRV	
Variable	M	SD	M	SD	Cohen's d	Effect size
FD	1.02	1.19	0.68	0.94	−0.32	*
F	8.92	5.34	9.69	5.12	0.15	
Pair	7.04	3.83	6.61	3.28	−0.12	
3r + (2)/R	0.38	0.16	0.35	0.14	−0.2	*
Lambda	0.86	0.95	0.92	0.85	0.07	
PureF%	0.39	0.17	0.42	0.18	0.17	
FM+m	4.87	2.89	4.67	2.75	−0.07	
EA	6.84	3.76	7.15	3.59	0.08	
es	9.09	5.04	8.57	5.14	−0.1	
D score	−0.68	1.48	−0.41	1.45	0.18	
Adj D	−0.2	1.23	0.09	1.17	0.24	*
a (active)	4.96	3.08	4.7	2.98	−0.09	
p (passive)	3.73	2.65	4.05	2.33	0.13	
Ma	2.09	1.83	2.06	1.81	−0.02	
Mp	1.67	1.61	1.93	1.47	0.17	
Intellect	2.35	2.57	2.98	2.59	0.24	*
Zf	12.5	4.92	12.84	5.65	0.06	
Zd	−0.67	4.72	−0.48	4.8	0.04	
Blends	4.01	2.97	3.75	3.12	−0.09	
Blends/R	0.18	0.13	0.17	0.14	−0.07	
Col-ShdBld	0.6	0.92	0.52	0.9	−0.09	
Afr	0.53	0.2	0.55	0.16	0.11	
Populars	5.36	1.84	5.22	2.02	−0.07	
XA%	0.79	0.11	0.78	0.12	−0.09	
WDA%	0.82	0.11	0.8	0.11	−0.18	
X+%	0.52	0.13	0.53	0.16	0.07	
X−%	0.19	0.11	0.19	0.11	0	
Xu%	0.27	0.11	0.25	0.12	−0.17	
Isolate/R	0.2	0.14	0.18	0.13	−0.15	
H	2.43	1.89	2.45	2.21	0.01	
(H)	1.22	1.24	0.92	0.96	−0.27	*
Hd	1.52	1.71	1.76	1.54	0.15	
(Hd)	0.64	0.92	0.85	0.95	0.22	*
Hx	0.41	0.98	0.34	0.83	−0.08	

(Continued on next page)

Table A3. (Continued)

Variable	International		England		England vs. CIRV	
	M	SD	M	SD	Cohen's d	Effect size
H + (H) + Hd + (Hd)	5.83	3.51	5.99	3.19	0.05	
A	7.71	3.18	8.09	3.16	0.12	
(A)	0.42	0.73	0.31	0.57	−0.17	
Ad	2.41	1.97	2.75	1.82	0.18	
(Ad)	0.16	0.45	0.17	0.41	0.02	
An	1.16	1.42	1.28	1.21	0.09	
Art	1.22	1.45	1.26	1.47	0.03	
Ay	0.52	0.87	1.17	1.26	0.6	**
Bl	0.25	0.55	0.27	0.58	0.04	
Bt	1.41	1.44	1.31	1.2	−0.08	
Cg	1.89	1.77	1.68	1.97	−0.11	
Cl	0.18	0.46	0.13	0.4	−0.12	
Ex	0.19	0.48	0.16	0.52	−0.06	
Fi	0.5	0.8	0.31	0.72	−0.25	*
Food	0.33	0.66	0.3	0.53	−0.05	
Ge	0.26	0.62	0.34	0.66	0.12	
Hh	0.84	1.03	1.23	1.4	0.32	*
Ls	0.87	1.12	0.95	1.2	0.07	
Na	0.75	1.11	0.74	1.29	−0.01	
Sc	1.11	1.35	1.67	1.66	0.37	*
Sx	0.47	0.94	0.59	0.97	0.13	
Xy	0.19	0.52	0.15	0.42	−0.08	
Idiographic	0.89	1.21	0.49	0.66	−0.41	*
DV	0.65	0.99	0.55	1.06	−0.1	
INCOM	0.73	0.97	0.92	0.91	0.2	*
DR	0.49	0.96	0.38	0.72	−0.13	
FABCOM	0.45	0.76	0.45	0.69	0	
DV2	0.01	0.14	0	0	−0.1	
INC2	0.1	0.33	0.2	0.53	0.23	*
DR2	0.06	0.31	0.01	0.11	−0.21	*
FAB2	0.08	0.31	0.24	0.57	0.35	*
ALOG	0.16	0.46	0.28	0.71	0.2	*
CONTAM	0.02	0.15	0.01	0.11	−0.08	
Sum 6 SpSc	2.75	2.39	3.05	2.64	0.12	

(Continued on next page)

Table A3. (Continued)

Variable	International		England		England vs. CIRV	
	M	SD	M	SD	Cohen's d	Effect size
Lvl 2 SpSc	0.25	0.62	0.45	0.79	0.28	*
WSum6	7.63	7.75	9.39	9.4	0.2	*
AB	0.32	0.82	0.27	0.69	−0.07	
AG	0.54	0.86	0.74	0.96	0.22	*
COP	1.07	1.18	1.28	1.23	0.17	
CP	0.02	0.15	0.01	0.11	−0.08	
Good HR	3.7	2.18	3.53	2.2	−0.08	
Poor HR	2.86	2.52	3.2	2.48	0.14	
MOR	1.26	1.43	1	1.16	−0.2	*
PER	0.75	1.12	0.25	0.61	−0.55	**
PSV	0.23	0.56	0.24	0.48	0.02	

Note. Effect size: *small (between 0.20 and 0.49), **medium (between 0.50 and 0.79).

Summary

This study provides Rorschach data for 88 adults aged 18–65 from the general population in England. We attempted to match our sample as closely as possible with census data on the variables of gender, age, marital status, ethnicity, geographical location, occupation, and level of education. For geographical location, we had too many participants in the South East and not enough in Yorkshire and the Midlands. This is a function of where the examiners were based. For education, we had too many educated participants. For occupation, we had too many unemployed participants and not enough in the semi-skilled category. For all other demographic variables, our sample is representative of the general population.

The Rorschach was administered according to the Comprehensive System by five experienced psychologists. Participants also completed a measure of psychological distress called the CORE. According to this measure, 20% of our participants were experiencing a clinically significant level of distress at the time when they took the Rorschach.

One quarter of the protocols were rescored to calculate interscorer reliability. This was found to be excellent for all variables apart from the six cognitive special scores, for which it was fair. Rorschach data are presented for Comprehensive System variables and compared with Exner's (2007) sample of 450 nonpatient adults in the United States and with the international reference sample (Meyer, Erdberg, & Shaffer, 2007). Number of responses was not significantly different. As compared with Exner's sample, we obtained large differences for eight variables, moderate differences for 28 variables, small differences for 43 variables, and no significant differences for 34 variables. Compared with the international reference sample, there were no large differences for any of the variables and a moderate difference on one variable only (Ay), with the English sample obtaining a higher mean. Our sample had lower form quality as compared with Exner's sample but it was in line with the international reference sample. Some other differences are discussed.

Résumé

Cette étude présente les données du Rorschach pour 88 adultes de 18 à 65 ans issus de la population générale de l'Angleterre. Nous avons tenté de former notre échantillon au plus près des données du recensement pour les variables genre, âge, statut marital, ethnicité, zone géographique, statut professionnel et niveau d'étude. Concernant les zones géographiques, nous avons trop de participants en provenance du Sud Est et pas assez en provenance du Yorkshire et des Midlands, en raison du lieu de résidence des examinateurs. Concernant le niveau d'étude, il est plus élevé que la moyenne, et nous avons trop de participants sans emploi et pas assez dans la catégorie intermédiaire. Pour toutes les autres variables démographiques, notre échantillon est représentatif de la population générale.

Le Rorschach a été administré selon les procédures du Système Intégré par cinq psychologues expérimentés. Les participants ont aussi complété une mesure de détresse psychologique appelée CORE. D'après cette mesure, 20% des participants présentaient un niveau cliniquement significatif de détresse au moment où ils ont passé le Rorschach.

Un quart des protocoles ont été re-cotés de manière indépendante et la fiabilité inter-correcteurs a été excellente pour toutes les variables à l'exception des six cotations spéciales cognitives où elle est satisfaisante. Les données des variables Rorschach en Système Intégré sont présentées et comparées d'une part avec l'échantillon d'Exner (2007) pour 450 adultes des Etats-Unis et d'autre part avec l'échantillon de référence international (Meyer, Erdberg, & Shaffer, 2007). Le nombre de réponses n'était pas significativement différent. Par rapport à l'échantillon d'Exner nous avons obtenu des différences importantes pour huit variables, modérées pour 28 variables, petites pour 43 variables et pas de différence pour 34 variables. Par rapport à l'échantillon de référence international, nous n'avons trouvé aucune différence importante, et une seule différence modérée pour la variable (Ay) qui est plus élevée dans l'échantillon anglais. Notre échantillon présentait une qualité formelle plus basse que dans l'échantillon d'Exner mais comparable avec celle de l'échantillon de référence international. Quelques autres différences sont discutées.

Resumen

Este estudio ofrece los datos de Rorschach de 88 adultos, de 18 a 65 años, de la población general de Inglaterra. Hemos tratado de ajustar lo mejor posible la muestra a los datos del censo en las variables de género, edad, estado civil, raza, procedencia geográfica, situación laboral y nivel educativo. No obstante, en cuanto a la procedencia geográfica, conseguimos muchos más participantes del Sureste y menos de Yorkshire y Midlands. Esto estuvo en función del lugar de residencia de los examinadores. En cuanto al nivel educativo, reunimos muchos más participantes de nivel alto. En cuanto a la situación laboral, tuvimos muchos más sujetos sin empleo y menos en la categoría de semicualificados. En todas las demás variables demográficas, la muestra es representativa de la población general.

El Rorschach se administró por parte de cinco psicólogos experimentados y siguiendo los criterios del Sistema Comprehensivo. Los participantes completaron también una medida de estrés psicológico llamada CORE. De acuerdo con esta medida, el *20% de los mismos estaban experimentando un nivel clínicamente significativo de estrés en el momento de su examen con Rorschach.*

Un cuarto de los protocolos se recodificó para calcular la fiabilidad inter-puntuadores. Ésta resultó ser excelente en todas las variables, excepto en los Seis Códigos Especiales cognitivos, en los que fue aceptable. Se presentan los datos de Rorschach para las variables del Sistema Comprehensivo y se comparan con los ofrecidos por Exner (2007) en una muestra de 450 adultos no-pacientes de Estados Unidos y con la muestra de referencia internacional (Meyer, Erdberg, y

Shaffer, 2007). El número de respuestas no ofrece diferencias significativas. En comparación con la muestra de Exner, nosotros obtenemos diferencias importantes en ocho variables, diferencias moderadas en 28 variables, pequeñas diferencias en 43 variables y ninguna diferencia en 34 variables. En comparación con la muestra de referencia internacional, no aparecen amplias diferencias en ninguna variable y encontramos una diferencia moderada en una sola variable (Ay), en la que la muestra inglesa obtiene una Media más alta. También observamos una Calidad Formal más baja en relación con la muestra de Exner, pero similar a la de la muestra de referencia internacional. Se discuten también algunas otras diferencias.

要約

ロールシャッハ包括システムにおける英国の標準研究

本研究は英国の一般人口における18-65歳の88人の成人のロールシャッハ・データを提供している。われわれは、性や年齢、婚姻状態、民族、地理的位置、職業、教育レベルを可能な限りマッチさせよう試みた。地理的な位置に関しては、サウス・イーストの参加者が非常に多く、ヨークシャーとミッドランドの参加者が十分ではなかった。これは検査者がどこに所在しているかに依っていた。教育に関しては、教育水準が高い参加者が多すぎた。職業について言えば、就業していない参加者が多すぎ、半熟練のカテゴリーに該当する参加者が十分でなかった。この他のすべての人口統計学的な変数については、われわれのデータは一般人口を代表していた。ロールシャッハは5名の経験豊富な心理学者によって包括システムによって施行された。参加者はまたCOREと呼ばれる心理学的な苦悩の尺度を完成させた。この尺度によれば、われわれの研究の参加者の20%がロールシャッハを受検した時に、臨床的に重篤なレベルの苦悩を経験していた。全プロトコルの4分の1が評定者間の信頼性を計算するために再スコアされた。この結果は、6つの認知の特殊スコアがまずまずであることをのぞけば、一致率は素晴らしいものであった。ロールシャッハ・データは包括システムの変数とされ、Exner's (2007)の米国における450名の非患者である成人データのサンプル、および国際的な比較サンプル（Meyer, Erdberg, & Shaffer, 2007）と比較された。反応数について有意差は認められなかった。Exnerのサンプルに比較して、われわれは8つの変数で大きな差異を、28の変数である程度の差異、43の変数で小さな差異を得たが、34の変数では有意差は見出されなかった。国際的な比較サンプルとの比較では、大きな差異を得た変数はなく、ある程度の差を一つの変数だけ（Ay）であり、これは英国のサンプルの方が高い平均が得られた。Exnerのサンプルに比較してわれわれのサンプルは形態水準が低かったが、国際的な比較サンプルには応じていた。他のいくつかの相違について考察をおこなった。

Research Article

Clients' TAT Interpersonal Decentering Predicts Psychotherapy Retention and Process

Sharon Rae Jenkins and Rachel B. Nowlin

Psychology Department, University of North Texas, Denton, TX, USA

Abstract: This naturalistic pilot study examined interpersonal decentering, a form of social cognitive maturity and self–other mentalizing scored from the Thematic Apperception Test, as a client personality variable that might predict psychotherapy retention and clients' perceptions of in-session process. Clients having difficulty with mature decentering might struggle to engage in therapy, need different interventions, and be at risk for therapy dropout. Thematic Apperception Test stories were gathered from new outpatient therapy clients soon after their intake session. Interpersonal decentering scores from the nine stories were used to predict outpatients' therapy attrition or perceptions of psychotherapy process four to six sessions later. Clients' perceptions of therapy events commonly associated differentially with psychodynamic and cognitive-behavioral therapies were measured using self-rated items from the Psychotherapy Process Q-set. Lower decentering scores predicted early attrition (before Session 6). Clients with more mature decentering scores reported more frequent psychodynamic relative to cognitive-behavioral therapy process events in these early sessions. Lower decentering maturity may limit clients' processing of psychodynamic interventions. Interpersonal decentering may be a valuable, easy-to-score assessment tool for predicting attrition risk and making treatment planning recommendations for intervention strategies.

Keywords: decentering, psychotherapy process, role-taking, Thematic Apperception Test, therapy dropout

One client characteristic that might predict therapy attrition or retention and shape evolving therapy process is the client's interpersonal skills and abilities, specifically transcendence of immature egocentrism in favor of mature understanding of other people's inner worlds of thoughts, feelings, intentions, and plans. Although social cognitive abilities normally develop in childhood and adolescence (e.g., decentering, perspective-taking, role-taking, mentalizing, theory of mind; Carpendale & Lewis, 2010), an adult's inclination to mobilize these abilities routinely is arguably a personality disposition that might be important in psychotherapy. Clients who consider more fully their therapist's intended meanings while deciding on their own responses to interventions seem less likely to misconstrue those interventions than are clients who take the therapist's words too concretely, all else equal.

Might clients who have difficulty mentalizing interpersonal interactions tend to drop out of therapy prematurely? Might such clients respond to various therapy processes differently from clients who have and use more mature relational capabilities? Might assessing social-cognitive maturity be helpful for treatment planning? Bram (2013) urged assessment psychologists to include measures of clients' relational capacities to make inferences and recommendations about the likely development of a good therapeutic alliance and how best to facilitate it for each client. Story-based assessment techniques can provide content-valid information about clients' social cognitive and narrative capacities with implications for psychotherapy (Jenkins, 2014).

The present study used a measure of interpersonal decentering to assess outpatient therapy clients' social cognitive maturity soon after intake in order to predict attrition from therapy and the clients' ratings of process events in therapy during the first six sessions.

Interpersonal Decentering

Of greatest interest for adult psychotherapy are the forms of social cognition among the latest to emerge developmentally as aspects of executive functioning, which have been called *perspective-taking*, *role-taking*, and *decentering* (Jenkins, Dobbs, & Leeper, 2015). These constructs converge at the understanding that social relationships go better when, before taking an action, a person considers the likelihood that other people's view of the world might differ from the person's own, thus transcending egocentrism to take the other's perspective or role. Considering the other person's possible thoughts, feelings, needs, intentions, and responses to one's action before acting should result in better interpersonal relations (Feffer & Suchotliff, 1966). Thus, this construct cluster constitutes the second dimension of mentalizing described by Ekeblad, Falkenström, and Holmqvist (2016), that of mentalizing about self and others.

Present-day work on mature social cognition and on what is now called *theory of mind* in very young children (Carpendale & Lewis, 2010) evolved from an earlier literature on children's role-taking. That line of research appears to have stalled after an extensive review by Enright and Lapsley (1980) concluded that measurement problems were responsible for the widespread inconsistent findings. More recent studies of adults have addressed this cluster of social-cognitive constructs from several disciplinary viewpoints with varying measurement methods, although most are self-report (e.g., Bernstein et al., 2015; Dimaggio et al., 2009; Gehlbach, Brinkworth, & Wang, 2012). However, self-report measures are prone to biases due to social desirability and format-specific method error variance (e.g., Brenner & DeLamater, 2016; Holtgraves, 2017).

Table 1. Developmental model of interpersonal decentering

Piaget's theory	Pre-operational	Concrete operations, sequential processing	Formal operations, simultaneous abstract processing
Feffer's theory	Undifferentiated	Differentiated with increasing concrete complexity	Differentiated and coordinated, with increasing abstract complexity
Operationalized in story scoring categories	Characters described as similar or alike	Sequential action–reaction exchanges (more turns)	Internalization of others (more nested perspectives)
Decentering scores	1	2–4	5–9

Feffer's interpersonal decentering (Feffer, Leeper, Dobbs, Jenkins, & Perez, 2008; Leeper, Dobbs, & Jenkins, 2008) is a content analysis scoring system for thematic apperceptive techniques and other narrative tasks (Jenkins, Austin, & Boals, 2013; Jenkins et al., 2015). *Mature decentering* is conceptualized as the tendency to mobilize internalized reflective thoughts about people's mental states when explaining their behavior (including one's own); for example, when telling stories to explain the actions of people in a series of pictures (Jenkins et al., 2015). This narrative measure of social cognitive maturity represents a state capacity and trait tendency to take multiple perspectives simultaneously and to consider the effect of one's own actions on others. Because it is scored from thematic apperceptive stories told about people pictured in different social situations (Feffer et al., 2008), it samples imaginative social thoughts, is not subject to the measurement method response biases common among self-report scales, and is not dependent on clients' self-insight or ability to articulate their experience. Grounded in developmental theory as described by Feffer (1959, 1970; Feffer & Suchotliff, 1966), the concept of interpersonal decentering bridges from Piaget's concrete operational perspective-taking to the mature mentalization capacity to see one's planned action from the other's viewpoint and one's own perspective simultaneously (see Table 1). As a narrative-based clinical assessment tool, it comports well with systems for narrative analysis of psychotherapy transcripts (e.g., Angus, Levitt, & Hardtke's [1999] Narrative Process Coding System).

Interpersonal decentering is a content-based scoring system for narrative material, and its content validity supports its interpretation as a measure of social cognitive reflective thought or mentalizing. It represents a short form of Feffer's Role Taking Task (RTT; Feffer, 1959), in which, like the film *Rashomon* (Kurosawa, 1950), participants were asked to tell stories about pictures of several people, then retell the story from each character's perspective. The more complex RTT scoring system identified the extent to which the resulting series of stories was both differentiated (showed distinct character perspectives) and coordinated (clearly about the same incident). By developing a system to score only the initial story, the original validation study for the Thematic Apperception Test (TAT) version used here (Feffer & Jahelka, 1968) supports its criterion validity as a strong correlate of the original RTT scores derived from the whole series of stories. Enright and Lapsley's (1980) massive literature review of children's role-taking measures summarized the RTT child literature. Studies in adults include that by Sommers (1984), who found that high RTT scorers reported more intimate disclosures to same-gender peers than low scorers did.

Previous studies of interpersonal decentering using the initial story system differentiated adolescents diagnosed with schizophrenia from those not so diagnosed (Strober, 1979), showing the theory-of-mind deficits typical of that disorder. Jenkins et al. (2015) distinguished violence perpetrators (who scored lower) from domestic violence survivors and other clinic clients with nonproblematic relationships. Applied to expressive writing intervention essays about stressful relational events, higher decentering scores were associated with evidence of activated relational information processing (use of more cognitive words, especially insight words) and more positive emotion words (Jenkins et al., 2013), these word counts being associated with improved health after relational losses (Pennebaker, Mayne, & Francis, 1997). As a measure of spontaneously mobilized mature social cognitive processes, decentering shows promise in relation to low egocentrism, psychological mindedness, and engagement in psychotherapy.

Interpersonal Decentering and Psychotherapy Dropout

Premature termination from psychotherapy is a significant concern in research and clinical settings that plagues randomized controlled therapy trials (RCTs). Meta-analyses show from 19% to 46% of clients do not complete treatment (Swift & Greenberg, 2012; Wierzbicki & Pekarik, 1993). Much of the research examining therapy dropout or premature termination has focused on aspects of the therapy itself (e.g., therapists' training and orientation, the setting and design of therapy) and the therapeutic alliance. When client factors are considered, demographics, level of dysfunction, and client satisfaction with the therapy or therapist are most often studied. Fewer studies have examined clients' personality characteristics, although Blatt produced a considerable body of work on dependency and self-criticism (e.g., Blatt & Felsen, 1993; Blatt & Zuroff, 2005; Blatt, Zuroff, Hawley, & Auerbach, 2009) and there is some work on attachment (Diener & Monroe, 2011; Eames & Roth, 2000).

Even fewer studies have focused on clients' ability to engage in therapy based on their psychological mindedness. Psychological mindedness can be defined as attunement to the processes of psychotherapy, specifically the ability to recognize psychological processes and patterns in one's life. Psychological mindedness is conceptually linked to interpersonal decentering, as both involve a client's ability to represent internally past or future interpersonal interactions in order to process them in therapy. Nixon, Jenkins, and Labrie (2011) found that a community sample of women higher in interpersonal decentering rated themselves higher in psychological mindedness on that scale of the California Psychological Inventory than did women who scored lower.

Several studies have shown that more psychologically minded clients are less likely to drop out of therapy prematurely. Piper, Joyce, McCallum, and Azim (1998) found psychological mindedness assessed by a video interpretation task was related to positive therapy outcomes. In a partial-hospitalization setting, lower psychological mindedness predicted premature dropout, while high psychological mindedness appeared to buffer against symptom chronicity in those who completed therapy (Tasca et al., 1999). Ratings of outpatients' insight into dynamic processes predicted treatment length, with greater insight predicting less likely attrition (Høglend, Engelstad, Sørbye, Heyerdahl, & Amlo, 1994). The depressed outpatients in the RCT of Ekeblad and colleagues (2016) who showed lower pretreatment mentalization capabilities were rated lower in working alliance by their therapists and had worse outcomes. The capacity for mature mentalization of self and others that is measured by decentering should facilitate clients' retention in psychotherapy.

Measuring Therapy Orientation Processes

New lines of research are beginning to explore the role of patient insight capability in selecting appropriate interventions (Lehmann et al., 2015). Lehmann and colleagues used the Shedler-Westen Assessment Procedure (SWAP) Insight Scale to predict the focus of specific therapist interventions in the third or fourth session of therapy. Higher therapist-rated client insight was related to therapists' discussion of similar patterns of relationships and experiences over time, a topic of particular interest in psychodynamic therapy (PDT) compared with cognitive-behavioral therapy (CBT; Jones & Pulos, 1993).

Clients' psychological mindedness and insight into relational patterns are both important elements of psychodynamic psychotherapy and constructs of interest for interpersonal decentering. Jenkins and colleagues (2013) found that expressive writing essays that scored higher in interpersonal decentering contained more insight words. Might clients who engaged more mature interpersonal decentering processes be more likely to notice and recall psychodynamic interventions than cognitive-behavioral ones? To answer this question, we measured the degree to which the heterogeneous therapist and supervisor orientations in our university training clinic (including PDT, CBT, acceptance and commitment, attachment-oriented, humanistic, existential, trauma-focused, and eclectic) produced in-session therapy processes that resembled the most basic features of psychodynamic relative to cognitive-behavioral orientation as reported by clients early in treatment.

The Present Study

To address the gap in research linking social-cognitive client personality variables to therapy dropout and perceived therapy process, we focused on the role of clients' interpersonal decentering. Mature decentering processes should provide better client relationship capabilities that in turn could enhance clients' understanding of the therapist's communications and insight into their own functioning, and thus their capacity to engage in the work of therapy, making early dropout less likely.

Further, owing to the attention paid to discussion of the therapy relationship in most psychodynamic therapies, we suspected that clients who began therapy with more mature decentering might engage more readily with the more exploratory, relational, and emotion-focused psychodynamic interventions than with the more cognitive, directive, and didactic cognitive-behavioral ones. This would result in such clients rating psychodynamic process events as more frequent than cognitive-behavioral ones. This could be attributable to more mature client decentering facilitating (a) clients' awareness of and ability to respond to psychodynamic interventions, (b) therapists' use of more psychodynamic interventions with clients who appear more insightful, or (c) both, regardless of therapists' avowed theoretical orientation. Conversely, clients less able to mentalize interpersonal processes maturely might be less able to process psychodynamic interventions, or might induce therapists to respond with more concrete and directive interventions. Such clients might find the whole psychotherapy process difficult, increasing risk of dropout.

Thus, we evaluated the role of clients' interpersonal decentering, measured soon after intake, as a (negative) predictor of early therapy attrition (i.e., within six sessions); and for retained clients, as a predictor of clients' perceptions of more frequent psychodynamic events (relative to cognitive-behavioral events). The following hypotheses were tested:

1. Less mature client decentering should predict early therapy dropout (by Session 6).

2. More mature client decentering should predict client's report of more psychodynamically oriented therapy events relative to cognitive-behavioral interventions by Session 6.

Method

Participants

Clients ($N = 47$, 30 women [63.8%] and 17 men [36.2%]) beginning therapy at a large public university's outpatient training clinic were recruited to participate. The clinic draws low-income individuals from the surrounding community, a small city in a rural region. The majority were Caucasian ($n = 35$; 74.5%); all others self-identified as African-American ($n = 12$; 25.5%). Ages ranged from 19 to 70 years ($M = 31.9$ years; $SD = 13.2$ years). Mean level of education was reported as "some college"; five participants (10.6%) held master's degrees, six participants (12.8%) held bachelor's degrees, 33 participants (70.2%) had some college or an associate's degree, and the remaining three participants (6.4%) had graduated high school, earned a GED, or less.

Measures

Interpersonal Decentering (Feffer et al., 2008)
The interpersonal decentering scoring manual assigns scores to participants' stories told about the TAT (Morgan & Murray, 1935) pictures (Cards 1, 2, 3BM, 4, 6BM, 7GF, 12 M, 13MF, and 10 were given in that order). Stories were narrated to the clinician, one of two advanced graduate students in the Clinical Psychology program, who wrote them down as verbatim as was feasible. They were typed organized by picture to facilitate consistent scoring. The scorer first reads the story and divides the narrative into interaction units, each involving the same characters interacting in the same location during the same period. Each unit is given one of nine maturity level scores representing increasingly complex differentiation and coordination of characters. These fall within two main levels of social information processing, concrete-sequential (scored 2–4) and internalized simultaneous (scored 5–9), which are both more mature than egocentric undifferentiation (scored 1). Higher scores indicate more frequent and complex interpersonal mentalization; lower scores show more preoccupation with back and forth action-reaction plotlines (see Tables 2 and 3 for examples). This summary is not adequate for attaining interscorer reliability; see Feffer et al. (2008). Details of scoring and examples are given elsewhere (Jenkins et al., 2015).

Table 2. Interpersonal decentering scoring categories

Score	Category description	Examples
1	Undifferentiated relationships	They went to the store together. Jose and Mariela got married.
2	Nonreactive directional relationships	The mother is looking at her daughter. George hated his boss.
3	Reactive directional relationships	Amber told Leon to leave; he ignored her. Harold punched his brother, who yelled.
4	Interactive directional relationships	Shonda asked her friend for the book, who gave it to her. She said, I'll return it Friday.
5	Internalized other, simple representation	Jacques was wondering about his wife. Ella wished she had a teacher.
6	Internalized other, surface characteristics	Joshua knew Brandy was a fast skater. Amanda expected that Mark would be late.
7	Internalized other, internalized state	Ana considered whether Joao would grieve. Ali didn't think Kesha loved him enough.
8	Internalized others	Veronica plans to surprise her daughter, who didn't know her father would be there.
9	Internalized self–other	Lily hopes she will be able to cheer him up. The coach regrets he made the boy play.

All stories were scored independently by both a master's-level graduate student and an advanced undergraduate psychology major who met regularly to compare their scores and reconcile discrepant scores. They were unaware of the follow-up measures or the present hypotheses and had been trained in using the Feffer et al. (2008) scoring manual for their own research. They had previously attained reliabilities exceeding .94 with expert scores on other stories. Interscorer reliability with consensus scores for all picture sets using Spearman's rho was above .90 (ranging from .92 to 1.00).

Three summary scores may be used depending on whether a maximal spontaneous performance (best effort, *state capacity*) or typical (traitlike *tendency*) performance across situations is needed (see Teglasi, Nebbergall, & Newman, 2012). The highest single score across all stories (best effort) shows the highest decentering maturity level the storyteller uses spontaneously, an estimate of decentering ability shown in the situations sampled by the pictures used (Jenkins, 2017b). The average of these highest scores for each story (*mean of highest*), shows how consistently across story situations the storyteller uses this highest level, estimating cross-situational generalizability versus situational specificity. Finally, the average score across interactions within each story, averaged across stories (*mean of means*), is interpretable as traitlike within-situation and cross-situational

Table 3. Two examples of interpersonal decentering scoring

Card 4. [*Wally wouldn't look her in the eyes*, not anymore. Her innocence, her naiveté, *they would all remind him of who he was not*. So he could brush her off,] (9) pull himself away, and go to work just like he did every day. [Laurie was always disappointed, "Why does he just brush me off, why won't he look me in the eyes?" She enjoyed *peering into the deep, calloused soul* of her husband.] (7) It had always been this way. She with the youthful smile, anticipating happiness, him ready to avoid it all. She had stopped trying to figure it out. [She just tried now to *figure out how to keep them both happy* together, without ever knowing who the other was.] (9) So this day was no different, [Wally shrugged her off and she wasted half of her morning *trying to answer why she would not grow resentful,* not grow bitter, she would continue to love him.] (9) But what happens the next time *[his glance floats her way* and he notices that the innocence is gone. Will he then be able to look into her eyes or will it be then that *he finally rejects her*?] (2, repeated, scored once)
Highest score = 9 Interaction Units = 5 Average = 36/5 = 7.2

Card 6BM. This woman's husband has just died and this is [someone *the doctor sent*] (3) to [come tell her. *He looks sorry and is sad to tell her* the news and she is in shock, denial.] (9) Then [*she will send him* away] (3) and [*call her son.*] (2)
Highest score = 9 Interaction Units = 4 Average = 17/4 = 4.25

Note. Interaction units are demarcated by brackets indicating changes in time, place, or person(s) present. Italic text indicates the phrase within an interaction unit that determines the decentering score. By convention, the first interaction in the second story is action–reaction: The doctor "sent" him, he responded by going. The same reasoning applies to the third interaction.

consistency. Because response productivity is the most common source of method error variance and validity threat for less structured data, both story length and number of interactions were correlated with each decentering score, revealing the need for statistically controlling for number of interactions in this study.

Therapy Orientation Process Scale (TOPS)
The TOPS items were taken from the Jones (1985) Psychotherapy Process Q-set from among those found empirically by Jones and Pulos (1993) to distinguish in-session events and behaviors more typical of PDT from those more typical of CBT. Jones and Pulos's clinical judges had classified each item into a nine-category Q sort forced normal distribution from 1 (least characteristic) to 9 (most characteristic). In the present study, clients rated each item on a 7-point scale ranging from *not at all* to *very much so*.

In their study of psychotherapy process measured from transcribed therapy sessions, Jones and Pulos (1993) applied the Psychotherapy Process Q-set to compare in-session processes of PDT and CBT. In their Table 4, Jones and Pulos listed the items that were most characteristic of and significantly differentiated CBT and brief PDT. We initially selected 22 items, 11 listed as most characteristic uniquely of each orientation, from Jones and Pulos's Table 4, given that each met the following criteria: (a) highly positively characteristic and not negatively (i.e., score

Table 4. Correlations of decentering scores with verbal fluency and clients' Therapy Orientation Process Scale (TOPS) ratings

	1	2	3[a]	4[a]	5	6
1. Mean N of interactions						
2. Mean N of words	.62**					
3. Decentering mean of highest[b]	.74**	.48**				
4. Decentering mean of means[c]	.26+	.15	.82**			
5. Psychodynamic (PDTS)	−.05	−.09	.14	.13		
6. Cognitive-behavioral (CBTS)	−.03	.04	−.06	−.04	.84**	
7. PDTS minus CBTS	−.04	−.22	.35*	.31+	.32*	−.24

Note. [a]Correlations in these columns have mean number of interactions controlled. [b]Highest Decentering score for each story, averaged across all stories. [c]Average Decentering score across all interaction units within each story, averaged across all stories. +$p < .10$. *$p < .05$. **$p < .001$.

closer to 9 than 1); (b) scores differed significantly between orientations; (c) the behavior or event is observable by both parties (i.e., not depending on inferences about either party's feelings, thoughts, or intentions); and (d) the language is accessible to the general public. Those requiring psychological sophistication or an understanding of therapy process, such as knowing what a *defensive maneuver* might be, were omitted or rephrased to common English (e.g., "T actively exerts control over the interaction [e.g., structuring, introducing new topics]" was rephrased to "Therapist actively directed the conversation."). The items are given in the Appendix.

Item reliability analysis was used to drop four items (of the 22 originally selected) having low item-total correlations, leaving 18 items for the final scale, nine for each subscale. Cronbach's α values were acceptable (Psychodynamic Subscale [PDTS]: α = .81; CBT Subscale [CBTS]: α = .80). The PDTS items' content centers on feelings ($n = 5$), relationships ($n = 2$), insight ($n = 1$), and repeating patterns ($n = 1$). The CBTS items' content focused on therapist directiveness ($n = 4$), ideas and reasoning ($n = 3$), therapist reassurance ($n = 1$), and use of humor ($n = 1$).

The two subscales correlated highly, $r = .85$, as expected given Jones and Pulos's (1993) explanation that the empirical differences they found are relative frequencies, not absolute discriminators. Thus, the individual scales share variance likely due to general therapist activity level creating more events of all kinds, and also to systematic error due to measurement method response sets for the rating scale. Therefore, the score of most interest is the relative PDTS difference score (PDTS minus CBTS), which controls for both sources of systematic error and represents the relative emphasis on psychodynamic processes compared with cognitive-behavioral processes as reported by clients. This difference score does not share the problems of difference scores used to measure change as reviewed by Gollwitzer, Christ, and Lemmer (2014).

Procedure

Participant data were gathered after approval by the university's institutional review board and the clinic's research review committee, and after each participant's informed consent was obtained. Participants were recruited by a letter of invitation included in the standard intake packet given to incoming clients who were identified as potential participants by their therapist with the supervisor's approval. Because therapists often did not identify potential participants until they had completed their first therapy session, some clients received the invitation letter when checking in for their second session. The letter described the study briefly and offered compensation of $15 for participation. The recruitment letter invited them to indicate consent to be contacted for participation in the study, which was done by checking a box and providing a signature on the form. Completed invitation letters were placed in the head researcher's clinic mailbox by office staff. The researcher then contacted these clients and gave more detailed information regarding the study's requirements and answered any questions clients had. If clients agreed to participate, an appointment was scheduled for the collection of Time 1 data. The researcher received written informed consent during that appointment. Clients were informed that participation was voluntary and not related to their ability to receive services at the clinic. They were also informed that the therapist did not know the details of the study or their participation, and they were asked to direct any questions about the study to the researcher.

At the first data collection session (Time 1, between intake and their third therapy session), clients first told stories about nine pictures, then completed demographic information and other self-report scales not used in this study. Time 2 data (TOPS) were collected four to six sessions after Time 1.

Results

Descriptive Analyses

Clients who dropped out by Session 6 ($n = 7$, 15%) were significantly younger than clients who stayed, $t(34.01) = -2.96$, $p = .006$. There were no significant differences in gender, ethnicity, or previous experience in therapy between dropouts and continuers.

Most of the variables were approximately normally distributed, except for best effort decentering scores (highest score across all stories), which had little variability; 44 (94%) of the sample attained at least one score of 9, and one each had a highest score of 2, 6, and 7. The client with the score of 2 also had an average number of interactions less than 1 per story (.78) and two stories with no interactions. Because this constitutes an inadequate data sample for this scoring system, this person was omitted from further analyses. Furthermore, the client who scored 6 dropped out, rendering best effort scores unsuitable for statistical analysis. Given that nine stories were gathered, sampling a good range of interpersonal situations (Jenkins, 2017b), these three scores, certainly the 2 and 6, suggest either deficient narrative capacity or serious social cognitive impairment for adults. This finding should inform future research.

Client demographics and therapy experience were not associated with the variables of interest. Decentering scores, dropout, and relative PDTS difference scores were all uncorrelated with client age, gender, educational level, number of children, number of past therapists, and total time in therapy.

Because response productivity is the major source of systematic method error for narrative techniques, associations of story length with scores were examined for possible control (McClelland, 1980). Further, for decentering, number of interactions provides a more relevant appraisal of response productivity because it captures an extraneous feature of narrative style, the preference for plotlines involving more changes of scene within a story, and is also highly correlated with story length, as shown in Table 4. With interactions controlled, correlation scores of story length with decentering best effort mean-of-highest and mean-of-means (average of within-story averages) dropped to $r = .04$ and $-.02$, respectively, and thus the remaining analyses were controlled for number of interactions.

Owing to the small sample size and the pilot nature of this study, α was set at $p < .10$.

Hypothesis Tests

1. Less mature client decentering should predict early therapy dropout (by Session Six).

With mean number of interaction units controlled for, low mean-of-means decentering scores were significant predictors of therapy dropout ($n = 7$). Clients who dropped out averaged 3.32 ($SD = 0.51$) on the 9-point scale, compared with those who remained, who averaged 4.0 ($SD = 0.98$). The resulting Cohen's d value (.79) represents a medium effect size, which was of acceptable significance, $F(1, 43) = 2.85$, $p = .10$, supporting Hypothesis 1. The finding was not significant for mean-of-highest scores, which averaged only the highest score for each story.

2. More mature client decentering should predict client's report of more psychodynamically oriented therapy process events relative to cognitive-behavioral events by Session 6.

With mean interactions controlled for, the mean-of-means decentering scores predicted relative PDTS difference scores toward the psychodynamic end, $r = .31$, $p < .07$. This correlation qualifies as a medium effect size of acceptable significance, supporting Hypothesis 2. Similarly controlled, the mean-of-highest finding, $r = .35$, $p < .04$, a medium effect size, also supported Hypothesis 2.

Discussion

This study produced two notable findings, both of medium effect size according to Cohen's (1992) classification. First, low decentering scores soon after intake predicted therapy attrition within six sessions. Second, more mature decentering predicted clients' reports of more frequent psychodynamic processes in session relative to cognitive-behavioral events. These results have implications for psychotherapy process and treatment planning.

Clients who typically presented concrete, specific, less mature decentering processing throughout their stories were less likely to continue therapy. Because mean-of-means scores are lowered by stories having more action–reaction interactions relative to mentalizing ones, this finding may reflect the departing clients' consistently greater storytelling interest in and involvement with concrete operations (action film plot lines) than with plots that demand more abstract thinking and concern with story characters' psychological processes. This is consistent with the findings that in general, psychological mindedness is related to both treatment completion (Tasca et al., 1999) and to better therapy outcomes across diverse therapy processes (Piper et al., 1998). Although some client attrition is likely due to variables unrelated to therapy process, consistent traitlike use of more mature social cognition appears to facilitate staying in therapy with novice therapists.

Perhaps our most useful finding is the prediction from decentering to client reports of relatively more PDT process events than CBT events. Multiple interpretations of these findings are possible. Objective ratings by trained observers might well have revealed differential emphasis on these interventions – or not. However, clients operating at a more mature decentering level might be more perceptive of PDT events than CBT processes. They might also find PDT techniques more emotionally engaging, and thus more memorable, than CBT techniques. Furthermore, such clients might process identical therapist statements in more psychodynamic ways than lower decentering clients do. Alternatively or concurrently, therapists who observed their mature-decentering client's greater psychological-mindedness might have chosen more PDT-style interventions because the client responded more favorably to those. Therapists of lower-scoring clients may have responded implicitly to their relatively lower insight by using more CBT interventions and fewer insight-leveraging ones that would have made demands on the clients' apparent deficits. If so, these clients perhaps experienced therapy as less daunting than otherwise, averting dropout. Finally, more psychologically minded clients might over time implicitly train their therapists in the direction of PDT interventions by their responsiveness to such, regardless of the therapist's specific treatment plan or stated orientation.

Strengths of the Study

This study has several important strengths. It is among few linking nonpathological aspects of client personality to psychotherapy dropout and therapy processes to improve treatment planning. If further research with larger samples supports the present findings, assessment psychologists may add interpersonal decentering to Bram's (2013) list of tools for evaluating clients' relational capacities relevant to attrition risk and recommending appropriate intervention strategies. This scoring system is efficient to score, can be scored reliably by undergraduate students, and can be integrated with other approaches to interpretation in multimethod assessment (Mihura & Graceffo, 2014).

The ecological validity of the study is high; given the heterogeneity of the client sample and therapist orientations, likely generalizability to similar training clinics is a strength. More experienced therapists might produce results with less random error variance. Finally, the effect sizes observed are quite respectable given that the hypotheses presented cross-method predictions, ruling out shared systematic measurement error that tends to inflate correlations among self-report scales (Hemphill, 2003).

Limitations of the Study

The major limitations of this study are its small sample size and its lack of systematic data on variables such as initial client diagnoses, symptom change, and specifics of clinicians' training and experience. Participating clients, being self-selected, might be more psychologically minded than most clients. Because dropouts could not be contacted to identify their reasons for leaving, we could not evaluate the accuracy of these interpretations. Because therapy process was measured via clients' perceptions of concrete session events, we cannot draw conclusions about therapists' intended intervention strategies, avowed orientation, or clients' responsiveness to these. However, the items of the Psychotherapy Process Q Set, including those chosen for the TOPS, are common to many orientations; the differentiation used here is a matter of relative balance among them based on Jones and Pulos (1993).

Future Research Needed

Future studies with larger samples and more experienced therapists should examine decentering, therapy process, clients' response to treatment, and measured therapeutic benefit over time. This includes studies of how clients' interpersonal decentering may interact with therapeutic techniques to enhance or limit the efficacy of different interventions while in therapy. More mature client decentering should predict greater engagement and benefit in therapies characterized by more psychodynamic processes. Conversely, clients who score in the impaired range might benefit more from CBT.

Measuring decentering processes in stories has the advantage of providing a congenial platform for intervention. Using a collaborative (Fischer, 1994) or therapeutic assessment approach (Finn, 2007), the clinician familiar with the Feffer et al. (2008) scoring system might test the limits after storytelling with an extended inquiry that provides increasing structure to scaffold a higher-level score (e.g., by asking, "What might this character be thinking? Does she know what he is planning to do? If she knows that, how would she decide how she should approach him next time?"). Such a story-mediated intervention strategy may be less taxing for low decentering clients than PDT interventions are, and thus perhaps less likely to increase attrition probability or weaken the alliance. Attending to the characteristics of the clients' response processes as they engage with our assessment tools (Annotti & Teglasi, 2017; Bornstein, 2011; Teglasi, 2013) can facilitate shaping our interventions to be organized similarly. Further discussion of the client's stories during the feedback session or in ongoing psychotherapy, and perhaps retelling some with direction from the therapist, could help a client become aware of the possible usefulness of decentering processes as tools for social understanding.

Acknowledgments

We thank Dr. Kristin (Niemeyer) Vaughn for allowing us to reanalyze her dissertation data for this project, Joshua A. Wilson for assistance with data analysis, and Dr. Summer Burkman and Mr. Luis Perez for scoring interpersonal decentering.

References

Angus, L., Levitt, H., & Hardtke, K. (1999). The Narrative Processes Coding System: Research applications and implications for psychotherapy practice. *Journal of Clinical Psychology, 55*(10), 1255–1270. https://doi.org/10.1002/(SICI)1097-4679(199910)55:10<1255::AID-JCLP7>3.0.CO;2-F

Annotti, L. A., & Teglasi, H. (2017). Functioning in the real world: Using storytelling to improve validity in the assessment of executive functions. *Journal of Personality Assessment, 99*, 254–264.

Bernstein, A., Hadash, Y., Lichtash, Y., Tanay, G., Shepherd, K., & Fresco, D. M. (2015). Decentering and related constructs: A critical review and metacognitive processes model. *Perspectives on Psychological Science, 10*(5), 599–617. https://doi.org/10.1177/1745691615594577

Blatt, S. J., & Felsen, I. (1993). Different kinds of folks may need different kinds of strokes: The effect of patients' characteristics on therapeutic process and outcome. *Psychotherapy Research, 3*(4), 245–259. https://doi.org/10.1080/10503309312331333829

Blatt, S. J., & Zuroff, D. C. (2005). Empirical evaluation of the assumptions in identifying evidence based treatments in mental health. *Clinical Psychology Review, 25*(4), 459–486. https://doi.org/10.1016/j.cpr.2005.03.001

Blatt, S. J., Zuroff, D. C., Hawley, L. L., & Auerbach, J. S. (2009). Predictors of sustained therapeutic change. *Psychotherapy Research, 20*(1), 37–54. https://doi.org/10.1080/10503300903121080

Bornstein, R. F. (2011). Toward a process-focused model of test score validity: Improving psychological assessment in science and practice. *Psychological Assessment, 23*(2), 532–544. https://doi.org/10.1037/a0022402

Bram, A. D. (2013). Psychological testing and treatment implications: We can say more. *Journal of Personality Assessment, 95*(4), 319–331. https://doi.org/10.1080/00223891.2012.736907

Brenner, P. S., & DeLamater, J. (2016). Measurement directiveness as a cause of response bias: Evidence from two survey experiments. *Sociological Methods & Research, 45*(2), 348–371. https://doi.org/10.1177/0049124114558630

Carpendale, J. M., & Lewis, C. (2010). The development of social understanding: A relational perspective. In W. F. Overton & R. M. Lerner (Eds.), *The handbook of life-span development, Vol 1: Cognition, biology, and methods* (pp. 584–627). Hoboken, NJ: John Wiley & Sons. https://doi.org/10.1002/9780470880166.hlsd001017

Cohen, J. (1992). A power primer. *Psychological Bulletin, 112*(1), 155–159. https://doi.org/10.1037/0033-2909.112.1.155

Diener, M. J., & Monroe, J. M. (2011). The relationship between adult attachment style and therapeutic alliance in individual psychotherapy: A meta-analytic review. *Psychotherapy, 48*(3), 237–248. https://doi.org/10.1037/a0022425

Dimaggio, G., Carcione, A., Nicolò, G., Conti, L., Fiore, D., & Pedone, R., . . . Semerari, A. (2009). Impaired decentration in personality disorder: A series of single cases analysed with the Metacognition Assessment Scale. *Clinical Psychology & Psychotherapy, 16*(5), 450–462. https://doi.org/10.1002/cpp.619

Eames, V., & Roth, A. (2000). Patient attachment orientation and the early working alliance: A study of patient and therapist reports of alliance quality and ruptures. *Psychotherapy Research, 10*(4), 421–434. https://doi.org/10.1093/ptr/10.4.421

Ekeblad, A., Falkenström, F., & Holmqvist, R. (2016). Reflective functioning as predictor of working alliance and outcome in the treatment of depression. *Journal of Consulting and Clinical Psychology, 84*(1), 67–78. https://doi.org/10.1037/ccp0000055

Enright, R. D., & Lapsley, D. K. (1980). Social role-taking: A review of the constructs, measures, and measurement properties. *Review of Educational Research, 50*(4), 647–674.

Feffer, M. H. (1959). The cognitive implications of role-taking behavior. *Journal of Personality, 27*, 152–158.

Feffer, M. (1970). Developmental analysis of interpersonal behavior. *Psychological Review, 77*(3), 197–214. https://doi.org/10.1037/h0029171

Feffer, M. H., & Jahelka, M. (1968). Implications of the decentering concept for the structuring of projective content. *Journal of Consulting and Clinical Psychology, 32*(4), 434–441.

Feffer, M., Leeper, M., Dobbs, L., Jenkins, S. R., & Perez, L. (2008). Scoring manual for Feffer's interpersonal decentering. In S. R. Jenkins (Ed.), *Handbook of clinical scoring systems for thematic apperceptive techniques* (pp. 157–180). Mahwah, NJ: Erlbaum.

Feffer, M., & Suchotliff, L. (1966). Decentering implications of social interactions. *Journal of Personality and Social Psychology, 4*(4), 415–422. https://doi.org/10.1037/h0023807

Finn, S. E. (2007). *In our clients' shoes: Theory and techniques of therapeutic assessment*. Mahwah, NJ: Erlbaum.

Fischer, C. T. (1994). *Individualizing psychological assessment*. Hillsdale, NJ: Erlbaum.

Gehlbach, H., Brinkworth, M. E., & Wang, M. (2012). The social perspective taking process: What motivates individuals to take another's perspective? *Teachers College Record, 114*(1), 1–29.

Gollwitzer, M., Christ, O., & Lemmer, G. (2014). Individual differences make a difference: On the use and the psychometric properties of difference scores in social psychology. *European Journal of Social Psychology, 44*(7), 673–682. https://doi.org/10.1002/ejsp.2042

Hemphill, J. F. (2003). Interpreting the magnitudes of correlation coefficients. *American Psychologist, 58*(1), 78–79. https://doi.org/10.1037/0003-066X.58.1.78

Høglend, P., Engelstad, V., Sørbye, Ø., Heyerdahl, O., & Amlo, S. (1994). The role of insight in exploratory psychodynamic psychotherapy. *British Journal of Medical Psychology, 67*(4), 305–316. https://doi.org/10.1111/j.2044-8341.1994.tb01799.x

Holtgraves, T. (2017). Social desirability and the interpretation of uncertainty terms in self-report questions. *Applied Cognitive Psychology, 31*, 623–631. https://doi.org/10.1002/acp.3364

Jenkins, S. R. (2014). Thematic apperceptive techniques inform a science of individuality. *Rorschachiana, 35*(2), 92–102. https://doi.org/10.1027/1192-5604/a000065

Jenkins, S. R. (2017a). The narrative arc of TATs: Introduction to the JPA special section on thematic apperceptive techniques. *Journal of Personality Assessment, 99*, 225–237. https://doi.org/10.1080/00223891.2016.1244066

Jenkins, S. R. (2017b). Not your same old story: New rules for thematic apperceptive techniques (TATs). *Journal of Personality Assessment, 99*, 238–253. https://doi.org/10.1080/00223891.2016.1248972

Jenkins, S. R., Austin, H., & Boals, A. (2013). Content analysis of expressive writing narratives about stressful relational events using interpersonal decentering. *Journal of Language and Social Psychology, 32*, 402–422. https://doi.org/10.1177/0261927X13479188

Jenkins, S. R., Dobbs, L., & Leeper, M. (2015). Using the Thematic Apperception Test to assess interpersonal decentering in violent relationships. *Rorschachiana, 36*, 156–179. https://doi.org/10.1027/1192-5604/a000064

Jones, E. E. (1985). *Manual for the psychotherapy process Q-set* Unpublished manuscript, University of California, Berkeley.

Jones, E. E., & Pulos, S. M. (1993). Comparing the process in psychodynamic and cognitive-behavioral therapies. *Journal of Consulting and Clinical Psychology, 61*(2), 306–316. https://doi.org/10.1037/0022-006X.61.2.306

Kurosawa, A. (1950). *Rashomon*. Tokyo, Japan: Daiei Film.

Leeper, M., Dobbs, L., & Jenkins, S. R. (2008). Melvin Feffer's interpersonal decentering. In S. R. Jenkins (Ed.), *Handbook of clinical scoring systems for thematic apperceptive techniques* (pp. 157–180). Mahwah, NJ: Erlbaum.

Lehmann, M. E., Levy, S. R., Hilsenroth, M. J., Weinberger, J., Fuertes, J., & Diener, M. J. (2015). Evaluating pretreatment patient insight as a factor in early therapeutic technique. *Journal of Psychotherapy Integration, 25*(3), 199–213. https://doi.org/10.1037/a0039560

McClelland, D. C. (1980). Motive dispositions: The merits of operant and respondent measures. In L. Wheeler (Ed.), *Review of personality and social psychology*. (Vol. 1). Beverly Hills, CA: Sage Publications.

Mihura, J. L., & Graceffo, R. A. (2014). Multimethod assessment and treatment planning. In C. J. Hopwood & R. F. Bornstein (Eds.), *Multimethod clinical assessment* (pp. 285–318). New York, NY: Guilford Press.

Morgan, C. D., & Murray, H. H. (1935). A method for investigating fantasies: The Thematic Apperception Test. *Archives of Neurology & Psychiatry, 34*, 289–306.

Nixon, J. A., Jenkins, S. R., & LaBrie, B. (2011, March). *TAT Interpersonal Decentering and social understanding*. Presented at the Society for Personality Assessment Annual Meeting, Boston, MA.

Pennebaker, J. W., Mayne, T. J., & Francis, M. E. (1997). Linguistic predictors of adaptive bereavement. *Journal of Personality and Social Psychology, 72*(4), 863–871. https://doi.org/10.1037/0022-3514.72.4.863

Piper, W. E., Joyce, A. S., McCallum, M., & Azim, H. F. (1998). Interpretive and supportive forms of psychotherapy and patient personality variables. *Journal of Consulting and Clinical Psychology, 66*(3), 558–567. https://doi.org/10.1037/0022-006X.66.3.558

Sommers, S. (1984). Social cognition and interpersonal affect: Correlates of role-taking skills in young adulthood. *The Journal of Genetic Psychology: Research and Theory on Human Development, 144*(2), 233–239. https://doi.org/10.1080/00221325.1984.9923429

Strober, M. (1979). The structuring of interpersonal relations in schizophrenic adolescents: A decentering analysis of Thematic Apperception Test stories. *Journal of Abnormal Child Psychology, 7*(3), 309–316.

Swift, J. K., & Greenberg, R. P. (2012). Premature discontinuation in adult psychotherapy: A meta-analysis. *Journal of Consulting and Clinical Psychology, 80*(4), 547–559. https://doi.org/10.1037/a0028226

Tasca, G. A., Balfour, L., Bissada, H., Busby, K., Conrad, G., & Cameron, P., . . . Turpin, P. (1999). Treatment completion and outcome in a partial hospitalization program: Interactions among patient variables. *Psychotherapy Research, 9*(2), 232–247. https://doi.org/10.1093/ptr/9.2.232

Teglasi, H. (2013). The scientific status of projective techniques as performance measures of personality. In D. H. Saklofske, C. R. Reynolds, & V. L. Schwean (Eds.), *The Oxford handbook of child psychological assessment (pp. 113–128). New York, NY: Oxford University Press.

Teglasi, H., Nebbergall, A. J., & Newman, D. (2012). Construct validity and case validity in assessment. *Psychological Assessment, 24*(2), 464–475. https://doi.org/10.1037/a0026012

Wierzbicki, M., & Pekarik, G. (1993). A meta-analysis of psychotherapy dropout. *Professional Psychology: Research and Practice, 24*(2), 190–195.

Received November 6, 2017
Revision received April 1, 2018
Accepted August 2, 2018
Published online November 9, 2018

Sharon Rae Jenkins
Psychology Department
University of North Texas
1155 Union Circle #311280
Denton, TX 76203-5017
USA
sharon.jenkins@unt.edu

Appendix

Therapy Orientation Process Scales (TOPS)

Directions: Below is a list of statements that describe things that therapists and clients do in psychotherapy. Think about the sessions you have completed and decide how much each statement describes your experience. Circle the number indicating your choice. [Scale range 1–7 anchored at "*not at all*" and "*very much so*"]

Psychodynamic subscale

5. (62) Your therapist identified a repeating pattern in your experience or conduct.
7. (32) You achieved a new understanding or insight.
9. (40) Your therapist shared his/her perceptions of your relationships with actual people in your life.
11. (50) Your therapist drew attention to feelings that you regard as unacceptable.
13. (22) Your therapist focused on your feelings of guilt.
15. (81) Your therapist emphasized your feelings to help you experience them more deeply.
17. (84) You expressed angry or aggressive feelings.
19. (92) Your feelings or perceptions were linked to situations or behavior of the past.
21. (100) Your therapist drew connections between your relationship with him/her and other relationships in your life.

CBT subscale

2. (38) There was discussion of specific activities or tasks for you to attempt outside of session.
4. (76) Your therapist suggested that you accept responsibility for your problems.
8. (27) Your therapist gave specific advice and guidance.
10. (30) Discussion centered on your ideas or beliefs.
12. (37) Your therapist behaved in a teacher-like manner.
14. (17) Your therapist actively directed the conversation.
16. (57) Your therapist explained the reasoning behind his/her technique or approach to treatment.
18. (66) Your therapist was directly reassuring.
20. (74) Humor was used.

Note. Items were selected from the Psychotherapy Process Q-set (Jones, 1985) based on analyses by Jones and Pulos (1993). Item numbers in parentheses are those of the original Q-set.

Summary

This naturalistic pilot study examined interpersonal decentering as a personality variable of patients that is scored from thematic apperceptive technique stories (TATs). This scoring system measures social cognitive maturity in children, adolescents, and adults. The study tested whether decentering scores would predict (a) the patient's continuation of psychotherapy, and (b) the patient's perceptions of psychotherapy process in the first six sessions of therapy.

The concept of decentering comes from Piaget's idea of perspective-taking in children. Melvin Feffer developed a scoring system for decentering (Feffer, Leeper, Dobbs, Jenkins, & Perez, 2008) that has nine levels of maturity, beginning with Piaget's concrete decentration. Feffer's system includes abstract, more mature levels that require evidence of internalization. The lower levels represent lack of differentiation of characters (scored 1) and concrete sequential processing represented by action–reaction statements (scored 2–4). The higher levels show abstract simultaneous processing requiring internalization (one character thinking about another person [scored 5–6], especially another person's internal experiences [scored 7–8], or contemplating the first character's own thoughts, feelings, or actions in relation to another [scored 9]). At its most mature level (9) decentering is a form of self-other mentalizing. Patients who do not show mature decentering might have difficulty engaging in therapy, might need different interventions, and might be at risk for therapy dropout.

TATs were gathered from new psychotherapy outpatients soon after their intake session. The nine stories were scored reliably for interpersonal decentering by an undergraduate student and a graduate student. These scores were used to predict (a) patients' therapy continuation or dropout and (b) patients' perceptions of the psychotherapy process after the first four to six sessions of therapy. Patients rated 18 items from the Psychotherapy Process Q-set (Jones, 1985) to describe what happened in the early sessions of therapy. Nine of these process events are more typical of psychodynamic therapy and nine are more typical of cognitive-behavioral therapy (Jones & Pulos, 1993). Scores were averaged for each therapy event type and the cognitive-behavioral average was subtracted from the psychodynamic average.

Lower decentering scores predicted dropout from therapy before Session 6. Patients with more mature decentering scores reported more psychodynamic therapy process events compared with cognitive-behavioral events up to Session 6. Lower decentering maturity might make patients at risk for dropout. Interpersonal decentering might be a valuable assessment tool for predicting risk of dropout and making treatment planning recommendations for therapy interventions.

Résumé

Cette étude pilote naturaliste a examiné le Décentration Interpersonnel comme une variable de personnalité des patients qui est notée à partir des histoires de technique d'aperception thématique (TAT). Ce système de notation mesure la maturité cognitive sociale chez les enfants, les adolescents et les adultes. L'étude a testé si les scores decentering prédisaient 1) la poursuite de la psychothérapie du patient, et 2) les perceptions du patient du processus de psychothérapie au cours des six premières séances de thérapie.

Le concept de décentration vient de l'idée de Piaget de la prise de perspective chez les enfants. Melvin Feffer a développé un système de notation pour decentering interpersonnel (Feffer, Leeper, Dobbs, Jenkins, & Perez, 2008) qui a neuf niveaux de maturité, en commençant par la décentration concrète de Piaget. Le système de Feffer comprend des niveaux abstraits, plus matures, qui nécessitent des preuves d'internalisation. Les patients qui ne présentent pas de décentration mûre pourraient avoir de la difficulté à s'engager dans une thérapie, pourraient nécessiter des interventions différentes et pourraient être à risque pour l'arrêt du traitement.

Des histoires de test d'aperception thématique ont été recueillies auprès de nouveaux patients externes en psychothérapie peu après leur séance d'admission. Les neuf histoires ont été notées de façon fiable pour Décentration Interpersonnel par un étudiant de premier cycle et un étudiant diplômé. Ces scores ont été utilisés pour prédire 1) la poursuite ou l'arrêt du traitement par les patients et 2) les perceptions des patients sur le processus de psychothérapie après les quatre à six premières séances de thérapie. Les patients ont évalué 18 items du Q-set du processus de psychothérapie (Jones, 1985) pour décrire ce qui s'est passé dans les premières séances de thérapie. Neuf de ces événements de processus sont plus typiques de la thérapie psychodynamique et neuf sont plus typiques de la thérapie cognitivo-comportementale (Jones et Pulos, 1993). Les scores ont été moyennés pour chaque type d'événement thérapeutique et la moyenne cognitivo-comportementale a été soustraite de la moyenne psychodynamique.

Les scores Décentration inférieurs prédisaient l'abandon du traitement avant la sixième séance. Les patients ayant des scores Décentration plus matures ont rapporté plus d'événements de processus de thérapie psychodynamique comparés aux événements cognitivo-comportementaux jusqu'à la sixième session. Décentration Interpersonnel pourrait être un outil d'évaluation précieux pour prédire le risque de l'arrêt du traitement et de faire des recommandations de planification de traitement pour les interventions thérapeutiques.

Resumen

Este estudio piloto naturalista examinó la decentración Interpersonal como una variable de personalidad de los pacientes que se puntúa a partir de historias de técnicas de apercepción temática (TAT). Este sistema de puntuación mide la madurez cognitiva social en niños, adolescentes y adultos. El estudio probó si las puntuaciones de Decentración Interpersonal predecían 1) la continuación de la psicoterapia del paciente, y 2) las percepciones del paciente sobre el proceso de psicoterapia en las primeras seis sesiones de terapia.

El concepto de descentramiento proviene de la idea de Piaget de la toma de perspectiva en los niños. Melvin Feffer desarrolló un sistema de puntuación para decentering (Feffer, Leeper, Dobbs, Jenkins y Perez, 2008) que tiene nueve niveles de madurez, comenzando con la descentración concreta de Piaget. El sistema de Feffer incluye niveles abstractos y más maduros que requieren evidencia de internalización. Los pacientes que no muestran Decentración madura pueden tener dificultades para participar en terapia, pueden necesitar diferentes intervenciones y pueden estar en riesgo de terapia abandonar.

Las historias de prueba de apercepción temática se recopilaron de nuevos pacientes ambulatorios de psicoterapia poco después de su sesión de admisión. Las nueve historias fueron calificadas de manera confiable para el decentering interpersonal por un estudiante de pregrado y un estudiante graduado. Estos puntajes se usaron para predecir 1) la continuación o el abandono de la terapia de los pacientes y 2) las percepciones de los pacientes sobre el proceso de psicoterapia después de las primeras cuatro a seis sesiones de terapia. Los pacientes calificaron 18 ítems del Q-set del Proceso de Psicoterapia (Jones, 1985) para describir lo que sucedió en las primeras sesiones de terapia. Nueve de estos eventos de proceso son más típicos de la terapia psicodinámica y nueve son más típicos de la terapia cognitivo-conductual (Jones y Pulos, 1993). Las puntuaciones se promediaron para cada tipo de evento de terapia y el promedio cognitivo-conductual se restó del promedio psicodinámico.

Los puntajes de Decentración inferior predijeron el abandono de la terapia antes de la sesión seis. Los pacientes con puntajes de descentramiento más maduros informaron más eventos del proceso de terapia psicodinámica en comparación con los eventos cognitivo-conductuales antes de la sexta sesión. La Decentración interpersonal podría ser una valiosa herramienta de evaluación para predecir el riesgo de dejar la terapia y hacer recomendaciones de planificación del tratamiento para las intervenciones terapéuticas.

要約

クライアントのTATの対人面における脱中心化は
心理療法の継続性とその過程を予測する

この自然主義的（原語：naturalistic）パイロットスタディは、TATでスコアされた患者のパーソナリティ変数のひとつとして対人関係における脱中心化を検討した。このスコアリングシステムは、児童、思春期、成人における社会的認知の成熟度を測定する。この研究では、脱中心化スコアが (a) 患者の心理療法の継続性 (b) セラピーの最初の6セッションにおける患者の心理療法過程に対しての捉え方（原語：perceptions）を予測できるかどうかを検討した。

脱中心化の概念は、ピアジェの認知発達理論に由来している。Melvin Feffer は、ピアジェの具体的操作期に見られる脱中心化から始まる成熟度を9段階からなる脱中心化スコアリングシステムを開発した（Feffer, Leeper, Dobbs, Jenkins, & Perez, 2008）。Fefferのシステムは、脱中心化の証拠が必要なより成熟したレベルである抽象的なもの（原語：abstract）が含まれている。より低いレベルであるスコア1は、キャラクターの未分化を表す。次に低いスコア2-4では、アクション—リアクションで表される連続的処理過程を具現化する。より高いレベルは、内在化を必要とする同時に起こるプロセスの抽象的なものを示す（他者のことを考えることができる人〔スコア5-6〕、特に他者の内的体験におけるものについてはスコア7-8、スコア9においては、他者との関係において、最初のキャラクターの思考、感情、活動について熟慮すること）。その最も成熟したレベル(9)では、脱中心化は、自他のメンタライジングの一形態である。成熟した脱中心化を示さない患者は、治療にのることが困難であり、他の違う介入を必要とするかもしれないし、心理療法からドロップアウトする可能性もあり得る。

インテイクセッションの後すぐに、心理療法の新規外来患者からTATは取られた。TATの9つの物語の中から対人面における脱中心化が、大学生と大学院生によってスコアされた。これらのスコアは、(a) 患者のセラピーの継続またはドロップアウト、(b) セラピーの最初の4から6セッションの後の心理療法過程における患者の捉え方を予測するために用いられた。患者はセラピーのはじめの方のセッションで、何が起こったかを記述するために、心理療法プロセスQセット(Jones, 1985)から18項目を評価した。これらのプロセス事象のうち9つは、精神力動的心理療法の最も典型的な例であった。そして9つは、認知行動療法の典型であった(Jones & Pulos, 1993)。各セラピーの事象タイプについてスコアの平均を出し、認知行動療法の平均から精神力動的心理療法の平均を差し引いた。

セッション6より前で、脱中心化指標が低く出た場合は、ドロップアウトを予測した。より成熟した脱中心化指標を示す患者には、セッション6までの認知行動療法よりも精神力動的療法の進展エピソードが多かった。脱中心化成熟度が低い場合には、ドロップアウトのリスクとなるであろう。対人面の脱中心化は、ドロップアウトのリスク評価、および心理療法介入についての計画提案の良いアセスメントツールであることが示唆された。

Research Article

Toward a Rorschach Hope Index

Anthony Scioli[1], Mike Cofrin[2], Friederika Aceto[3], and Timothy Martin[4]

[1]Department of Psychology, Keene State College, Keene, NH, USA
[2]Management in International Business, University of Applied Management Studies, Mannheim, Germany
[3]Private Practice, Boston, MA, USA
[4]Child and Family Psychological Services, Boston, MA, USA

Abstract: In this study, we derive a measure of hope from the Rorschach. Drawing on an integrative approach to hope, we identify six Rorschach variables, representing two dimensions each of: interpersonal perceptions, coping resources, and goal engagement. We empirically validate these variables against theoretically linked measures of attachment, coping, and mastery. We propose a Rorschach State Hope Index. To illustrate one potential benefit of this new measure, we apply the Hope Index retrospectively to an individual who died by suicide despite a relatively low score on the existing Suicide Constellation of the Comprehensive System.

Keywords: hope, hopelessness, suicide

For centuries, artists, scholars, and scientists have acknowledged the centrality of hope. Goethe dubbed it "[hope] a second soul" (http://m.notable-quotes.com/g/goethe_quotes_ii.html). Dostoyevsky wrote, "To live without hope is to cease to live" (http://www.wisdomquotes.com/quote/fyodor-dostoyevsky-2.html). Menninger (1959) believed hope was the "indispensable flame" of psychiatry and the "major weapon" against suicide. Jerome Frank (1974) distilled the "common factor" of hope from a quarter century of psychotherapy outcome research. In the laboratory, investigators are unearthing links between positive emotions such as hope and various health-related outcomes, from diet and physical activity to immune status and survival time in the presence of advanced cancer (Gottschalk, 1985; Scioli, MacNeil, Partridge, Tinker, & Hawkins, 2012; Scioli, Scioli-Salter, Sykes, Anderson, & Fedele, 2016). By comparison, hopelessness is associated with an assortment of human problems including capitulation in the context of serious illness, failures in the classroom and the workplace (Snyder et al., 1991), as well as depression and suicide (Abramson, Metalsky, & Alloy, 1989; Franklin et al., 2017; Kovacs, Beck, & Wiessman, 1975).

Historically, theories of hope emphasize one or more of the following: attachment resources (Erikson, 1950), coping strategies (Breznitz, 1986), or goal pursuits

(Stotland, 1969). Philosophers and theologians stress trust and community (Marcel, 1962/1944; Lynch, 1965). In nursing and medicine, the buffering benefits of hope are highlighted (Dufault & Martocchio, 1985; Nowotny, 1989). Psychologists focus on perceived goal success or agency (e.g., Stotland, 1969; Snyder et al., 1991). Unfortunately, current assessment tools rarely capture more than one or two of these hope dimensions. The widely used Beck Hopelessness Scale (Beck, Steer, & Brown, 1996) taps perceptions of future achievement success or failure. The Hope Scale (Snyder et al., 1991) addresses perceived agency and pathways toward goals. To advance the science and practice of hope, a broader assessment model is warranted.

Focus: Deriving Hope From the Rorschach

The Rorschach is one of the most widely used psychological tests in the world, providing a wealth of information regarding an individual's functioning. Neither Rorschach nor his immediate followers could have anticipated the development of an Egocentricity Index, a Depression Index, or a Suicide Constellation, all part of the current Comprehensive System (Exner, 2003). With respect to hope, we can presently derive perceptions of the interpersonal world (attachment), coping resources (survival), and goal engagement (mastery). In short, the raw elements for capturing hope already exist. If these elements can be extracted or adapted from widely known Rorschach variables, such as those present in the Comprehensive System (Exner, 2003), hope becomes immediately accessible to a great number of researchers and practitioners.

The present study is an outgrowth of an ongoing program to develop applications from an integrative theory of fundamental hope (Scioli & Biller, 2009; Scioli, Ricci, Nyugen, & Scioli, 2011). Philosophers generally distinguish ultimate hopes from fundamental hope (see Godfrey, 1987). Whereas ultimate hopes refer to specific aims, subject to endless revision in the course of a lifetime, fundamental hope is a character trait. In common language, we might equate it to *hopefulness* or what Erikson (1950) labeled *basic hope*. Scioli and Biller (2009) liken fundamental hope to an emotional network:

> We define [fundamental] hope as a future-directed, four-channel emotion network, constructed from biological, psychological, and social resources. The four constituent channels (dimensions) are the mastery, attachment, survival, and spiritual systems (or sub-networks). The hope network is designed to regulate these systems via both feed-forward (expansion) and feedback processes (maintenance) that generate a perceived probability of adequate power and presence as well as protection and liberation. (p. 30)

This conceptual foundation [of fundamental hope] guided the selection of six Rorschach variables, two variables each, for three of the four hope components – mastery, attachment, and survival. (At this time, we have set aside the fourth dimension of spirituality for future Rorschach studies.) We view fundamental hope as one emotion, albeit with multiple dimensions. This suggests the development of an index rather than a constellation. The former (index) preserves the notion of a singular construct whereas the latter, broader concept (constellation) subsumes multiple levels of elements, including one or more indexes as well as single determinants, ratios, and other derivations. (The nearest analogue is the Depression Index.)

To provide a greater context for the selection of the Rorschach variables, we briefly elaborate on the behavioral elements of hope in terms of attachment, survival, and mastery.

The Behavioral Elements of Hope and Hopelessness

A review of the literature reveals the following behavioral elements of hope and hopelessness:

Presence or Absence of Interpersonal Resources (Attachment)
To quote Pruyser (1987, p. 467) hope involves "a belief that there is some benevolent disposition toward oneself somewhere in the universe." In Erikson's (1950) developmental model, basic hope is a virtue derived from early trust experiences nurtured by a predictable caregiver. Lynch (1965) specifically rejected the notion of hope as a private resource and traced its origin to experiences of collaborative mutuality. Durkheim (1951/1897) linked despair and suicide to a lack of social integration (egoistic), group over-identification (altruistic), or the absence of social direction (anomic). Gabriel Marcel associated hopelessness with "the rupture of all living communications with others" (cited in Lester, 1995, p. 95). In a recent study, the risk of suicide was greatest among individuals who reported high levels of hopelessness as well as feelings of thwarted belongingness or perceived burdensomeness (Hagan, Podlogar, Chu, & Joiner, 2015).

Coping Resources or Deficits
Hopeful individuals possess a robust reality negotiation system that includes widescope primary appraisal processes (initial assessments of stressors) and a reflexively iterative secondary appraisal process (ongoing stress responses) that continually generates possibilities for improvement, recovery, or escape. Along

these lines, Folkman (2010) notes that hope, unlike denial or blind optimism, is a unique stress management process in facilitating a simultaneous intake of both positive and negative aspects of reality. Agreeing, Breznitz (1986) contends that hope does not involve a denial of reality but an enlarged perspective. In a classic study, Wright and Shontz (1968) identified the strategies of reality construction and reality surveillance that sustained hope in parents of children with life-threatening disabilities. The hopeless individual lacks these coping resources. Internal and external demands exceed one's capacity to generate a better outlook. The loss of hope creates tunnel vision, and the belief that no viable options remain (Beck, 1976). The classic representation of hopelessness from antiquity to the presence involves some form of entrapment; an individual bound with chains, buried alive, or adrift at sea (cf. Rosen, 1971; history of suicide).

Engagement With Life Goals (Mastery)
Descending from Mowrer (1960) and Stotland (1969), there is a tradition in psychiatry, and even more so within psychology, of equating hope with estimations of reward or goal attainment. Putting aside ultimate hope, the concept of fundamental hope also presumes an element of purpose, engagement, and persistence. This is evident in ancient passages (e.g., Aristotle's "Hope is a waking dream"; http://www.quotationspage.com/quote/24223.html) as well as in Bloch's (1986) modern eschatology of hope. Loss of motivation is one of three factors extracted from the Beck Hopelessness Scale (Beck, Weissman, Lester, & Trexler, 1974). The assessment of agency and pathways toward goals is the focus of the Snyder Hope Scale (Snyder et al., 1991). Scores on the Snyder measure relate to the establishment and pursuit of goals as well as performance attitudes, particularly in healthy young adults (Rand, 2009; Snyder et al., 1991). Scioli et al. (2011) found a strong correlation between the Mastery subscale of their Comprehensive Hope Scale and the NEO Achievement measure ($r = .51$, $p < .01$). By contrast, hopelessness involves the perception that one's goals are out of reach, and further efforts are futile (Abramson et al., 1989; Stotland, 1969). Forintos, Rózsa, Pilling, and Kopp (2013) showed that hopelessness correlates positively with a lack of life goals and negatively with perceived self-sufficiency. There is also evidence that low hope individuals may retain goals that are simultaneously seen as unattainable (Coughlan, Tata, & MacLeod, 2017; Hadley & MacLeod, 2010).

Rorschach Hope Variables

An analysis of Exner's (2003) Comprehensive System suggested the following six variables are candidates for deriving a measure of hope, as operationalized in the previous section (see Table 1).

Table 1. The Rorschach Hope Index

Dimensions of hope (Scioli et al., 2011)[a]	Hypothesized Rorschach variables
Attachment hope	
Trust	Good human representations
Connectedness and collaboration	Cooperative movement
Survival hope	
Positive appraisal system (+ coping bias & persistence)	Raw D (resources – demands)
Liberation beliefs and option building strategies	Active plus passive movement
Mastery hope	
Ambition and ideals	W:M (aspiration index)
Exploratory drive	ZSum

Note. [a]We exclude the fourth dimension of spirituality in the hope model from this research.

Presence of Interpersonal Resources (Attachment)
The perception of humans has been associated with interest in other people and the extent to which a person identifies with their social environment (Exner, 2003). What may be more relevant in the case of hope is the degree to which human percepts are positive or negative, benign or toxic. In the Comprehensive System, a scoring of *Good Human Representations (GHR)* involves percepts with an absence of negative indicators such as aggressive or morbid content as well those devoid of special scores, indicating serious cognitive or perceptual disturbances. One expects hopeful individuals to feel more positively connected to others, and to have healthier object representations. Such protocols should have significantly fewer human contents contaminated with negative markers.

The *cooperative movement* variable (perception of two or more objects interacting in a positive or collaborative manner) has been associated with perceptions of positive interactions among people and a willingness to participate in such interactions (Exner, 2003). Hopeful individuals demonstrate a greater tendency to imagine cooperative activities than those who are in a hopeless state. Lynch (1965) described the relational fabric of hope in terms of collaborative mutuality. Pruyser (1987) emphasized that in the experience of hope, as opposed to a state of optimism, individuals do not experience the ego as a solitary center of action.

The hypothesis tested in this study is whether good human representations and discernment of cooperative movement relate (respectively) to measures of interpersonal trust and a balanced engagement with life events (reliance on self *and* others).

Coping Resources (Survival)

The *D score,* sometimes labeled a *Stress Tolerance Index* (Exner, 2003) derives from the Experience Actual (EA) minus the es (Experienced Stimulation) variables. EA is the sum of Human Movement Responses and weighted chromatic color responses. The EA variable represents the volume, capacity, or storehouse of deliberate, ego-dominated coping resources. The es score is the sum of nonhuman responses plus shading, and reflects unorganized stimulus demands operating on the individual. A number of studies have shown that EA is greater in nonpatients than among patients, and that insight-oriented psychotherapy tends to increase both of the EA components while lowering es values (Exner, 1992; Exner, 2003). The Raw *D* score (EA – es) reflects the current capacity for managing stress and adequate self-regulation. Within the Comprehensive System, further computations are possible to produce adjusted es and adjusted *D* scores. However, these yield more trait-like variables whereas the present focus is on current levels of hopefulness. We also prefer the raw *D* score instead of the typical scaled *D* variable because the latter reduces variance by approximately one third (e.g., raw scores of +13 to +15 = a scaled *D* score of +5). The scaled *D* places more weight on the balance between EA and es as well as deviations from normative samples. By contrast, raw *D* scores should provide a purer measure of interindividual level, coping-related psychic resources versus demands. The first coping-related hypothesis tested in this study is whether the raw *D* variable relates to a positive view of the self as a capable, resilient individual.

Active Movement responses signify more deliberate and direct forms of coping, while *Passive Movement* responses suggest more indirect or delayed coping strategies. In the Comprehensive System (Exner, 2003) as well as in the stress and coping literature there has been a greater value placed on active coping strategies (Folkman & Lazarus, 1985). Nevertheless, indirect forms of coping are not necessarily maladaptive. In a classic review, DeGroot, Boeke, Bonke, and Passchier (1997) found that indirect forms of coping, including blunting and avoidance, might be more adaptive for short-term management of situations in which an individual is unable to exert much direct control. There are also cultural differences in preferred modes of control. Rothbaum, Weisz, and Snyder (1982) distinguish primary control from secondary control processes. The latter refers to indirect forms of influence that are typically favored in various non-Western countries, including many Asian cultures. There can be forms of delay, blunting, or fantasying, that are adaptive, not reducible to denial, and which may productively sustain the hoping process. The early Christian writer Tertullian described hoping as "patience with the lamp lit" (http://www.quotes-inspirational.com/quote/hope-patience-lamp-lit-48/). In summary, hope may incorporate both active and passive modes of coping. The second coping-related hypothesis is that the sum of Rorschach variables

Active Movement and Passive Movement relates to a standard measure of diversity in ways of coping.

Goal Engagement (Mastery)

The ratio of whole responses to movement responses (W:M) is an aspirational index that contrasts the level of perceptual effort (W) with the functional capabilities needed for achievement-oriented activities (M). *The weighted sum score of organized responses (ZSum)* is an index of organizational synthesis or perceptual complexity, revealing the extent to which an individual is motivated and able to integrate potentially disparate elements of a stimulus field. The perception of whole responses and the organization of blot elements require more work than a simple identification of unrelated elements. Both variables (W:M and ZSum) reflect the degree of psychological investment in a stimulus field (Exner, 2003). LaBarbera and Cornsweet (1985) identified ZSum as the strongest predictor in a discriminant equation used to distinguish children who improved during psychotherapy from those who regressed.

Breznitz (1986) suggested that hope brings an enlarged view of reality rather than a denial of the truth. Lynch (1965, p. 200) agreed and added, "The higher it [hope] would soar, the deeper [into reality] it must plunge." The hypothesis tested in this study is whether the W:M and ZSum variables relate to performance on a classic behavioral measure of goal engagement (an unsolvable puzzle task), and a measure of perceived agency.

A meta-analysis of Rorschach variables by Mihura, Meyer, Dumitrascu, and Bombel (2013) indicated good or excellent validity results for four of the six variables under investigation. The authors found little or no data to support ZSum or W: M as indicators of processing investment or aspiration. Czopp and Zeligman (2016) challenged these conclusions, arguing that Mihura et al. applied overly narrow study selection criteria. (We also note that Mihura et al. did not report negative findings related to either variable.) By contrast, Exner (2003) made a strong logical and theoretical argument for including both variables in the assessment process. Both variables remain in the structural summary of the Comprehensive System. This collection of factors further highlights the need to evaluate whether ZSum and W:M scores correlate with established measures of goal engagement.

Method

Subjects and Procedure

The participants were 25 students recruited from psychology classes at a public liberal arts college in the Northeastern United States. The mean age for this sample was 19.26 years and included eight males and 17 females. All participants were individually tested. Two graduate students, trained in the Exner (2003) system, and blind to other test results, administered the Rorschach. Subsequently, the participants worked on a puzzle task (a measure of goal engagement, described in the next section), followed by a brief demographics form and several questionnaires to address interpersonal perceptions, coping resources, and goal engagement.

Validation Measures

The Rotter Interpersonal Trust Scale is a 40-item self-report instrument (25 trust; 15 filler items) for the assessment of generalized trust in others (Rotter, 1967). The Trust Scale has been validated against self-reports, peer ratings, and in laboratory settings. In this study, we used a reduced 15-item version of this scale based on a factor analysis conducted with four large samples of young adults, similar in age to the participants in this present research (Wright & Tedeschi, 1975). This young adult version taps paternal and political trust as well as trust in strangers. The α value computed in the present sample was .75.

The Ways of Coping – Revised (WOC; Folkman & Lazarus, 1985) is a 66-item questionnaire for assessing an individual's reported use of different coping strategies. The full instrument contains eight scales. In this study, we created a brief coping measure by combining three of the first four scales (Scale 1: Problem-Solving; Scale 2: Wishful Thinking; and Scale 4: Seeking Social Support). Statistically, these scales have shown the strongest reliability (α = .88, .86, and .82, respectively). Conceptually and collectively, they represent two alternative, direct ways of coping (problem-solving and social support) and one indirect manner of coping (wishful thinking). The content of the third scale encompasses more than wishful thinking and includes references to use of fantasy and imagination. The three scales formed an internally consistent whole (sample α = .80). To validate the Rorschach attachment-related variable of Cooperative Movement, we derived a self versus other balance score by subtracting Social Support WOC from Problem-Solving WOC and subsequently computing Z and T-score transformations. In the resulting distribution, higher scores represent greater balance (reduced differences between self and other WOC). In addition, we used the brief WOC total score to validate the Rorschach-derived coping variable (Active plus Passive Movement).

The Cognitive Triad Index (CTI; Beckham, Leber, Watkins, Boyer, & Cook, 1986) draws on Beck's triadic theory of depression. The authors created three CTI subscales, of 10 items each, tapping perceptions regarding the self, the world, and the future. The total CTI score correlates strongly with self-reported and clinical ratings of depression. Subsequent factor analyses of young adults reveal five factors (Anderson & Skidmore, 1995). We selected Factor 3 because it most resembled a resiliency factor, consisting primarily of positive views regarding the self, including the following items: "I am as adequate as other people I know" (17), "I can do a lot of things well" (25), "I can't do anything right" (13, reverse-scored). The other four factors consisted of world or future items (Factors 1, 2, and 4), or negatively worded self items mixed with future items (Factor 5).

The classic puzzle task developed by Glass and Singer (1972) includes solvable and unsolvable puzzles. This task set has appeared in studies of achievement and stress tolerance for nearly three decades. The objective is to trace a puzzle without retracing any lines or lifting the writing instrument from the paper. In this study, we employed one solvable and one unsolvable puzzle. Participants had 5 min to solve each puzzle, and then allowed extra time to continue working on the problem, unless they wished to stop. Nearly every participant took advantage of the extra-time offer. (There were no Rorschach-related differences in number of participants opting for extra time.) The solvable puzzle is merely an introduction to the real task. The dependent variable is the number of attempts made on the unsolvable puzzle task.

The Hope Scale (Snyder et al., 1991) is a 12-item self-report measure of trait hope. Four are filler items; four items represent agency (self-efficacy), and four items represent perceived pathways toward goals. In previous studies, Snyder et al. (1991) have demonstrated the reliability and validity of the hope scale. Typical α values for agency and pathways range from .71 to .76 and .63 to .80, respectively. The total internal validity of the Hope Scale ranges from .74 to .84. Individuals who score higher on the Hope Scale report better college grades and set difficult goals (Snyder et al., 1991). While not considered a comprehensive measure, the Hope Scale captures a dimension of self-efficacy (Agency) that is theoretically relatable to the ZSum (input or processing motivation) variable, particularly if we accept the classic insights of White (1959, p. 330), who conceptualized mastery in terms of an exploratory and experimental attitude, a "steady persistent inclination toward interacting with the environment." In this study, we used only the Agency subscale.

Results

Interrater Reliability

Two graduate students trained in the Exner system and blind to each other's results scored the first 20 protocols (80%). The level of agreement for the six variables ranged from 80% to 95%. The overall level of agreement was 86% (103/120).

Correlates of the Hope Index
There were no age or gender differences. The Hope Index (total score, 0–6) showed little redundancy with the Exner Depression Index ($r = -.17$, $p > .05$) or the Suicide Constellation ($r = .18$, $p > .05$). We discuss these relationships later in this article.

Construct Validation of Rorschach Hope Variables

We divided five of the six Rorschach variables into low, medium, and high values. We did this for two reasons. Many Rorschach variables reveal a skewed distribution, with data clusters interrupted by one or more outliers, making correlational analyses difficult, if not misleading. Secondly, the creation of levels may provide future guidelines for potential cutoff scores, especially when compared with existing norms (Exner, 2003). One exception was the Cooperative Movement variable where the distribution (0 or higher) necessitated a medium split into low and high values.

Each of the six Rorschach variables demonstrated a significant relationship with theoretically linked measures of hope elements. The results in Tables 1, Table 2, and Table 3 include group sample sizes (by levels of Rorschach variables), means, and standard deviations. We present t values for all significant group differences and reference Exner (2003) norms for comparison. We include effect sizes (Cohen's d), which ranged from .86 to 1.51; Cohen (1988) designated effect sizes > .80 as indicative of large or clearly perceptible laboratory differences.

In Table 2, we display the results for the attachment variables. Participants with Rorschach protocols containing four to seven Good Human Representations (GHR) scored significantly higher on the Rotter Interpersonal Trust Scale, $t(18) = 2.40$, $p < .05$, as compared with those with one to three GHR. Individuals with more than seven GHR and those with four to seven GHR did not differ in trust. Participants with at least one Cooperative Movement response scored significantly higher on a measure of balanced coping (self-reliance vs. social support): $t(23) = 2.19$, $p < .05$.

Results for the coping variables appear in Table 3. Individuals with raw D scores greater than 2.50 demonstrated significantly higher scores on the resiliency factor of the Cognitive Triad Index as compared with those with negative values: $t(14) = 3.01$, $p < .01$. Those with raw D scores of 0–2.50 also showed a trend toward higher resiliency scores as compared with those with negative

Table 2. Construct validation of Rorschach Hope Index variables: attachment hope

	Rotter Interpersonal Trust Scale		
		Trust Score	
	N	M	SD
Good human representations[a]			
(1.00–3.00) Low	7	37.50	3.73
(4.00–7.00) Medium	13	41.95	4.05
(8.00–12.00) High	5	41.60	6.80
Low vs. medium: $t(18) = 2.40$, $p < .05$ (Cohen's d effect size = 1.14)			

	Ways of Coping Scale (WOC)		
		Self vs. Other Balance Score[b]	
	N	M	SD
Cooperative movement[c]			
(0.00) Low	14	41.79	11.29
(1.00–3.00) High	11	50.00	5.80
Low vs. high: $t(23) = 2.19$, $p < .05$ (Cohen's d effect size = .96)			

Note. [a]Mean of Exner (2003): Extratensives and introversives = 5.31. [b]Z and T-score transformations of Problem-Solving WOC (self-reliance) minus Social Support WOC. Higher values represent a more even balance of reliance on self and others. [c]Mean of Exner (2003): Extratensives and introversives = 2.14.

values: $t(16) = 1.82$, $p = .08$. Participants whose Active + Passive Movement sum was 10 or higher had significantly higher scores on the Ways of Coping (total) scale as compared with those whose Movement sum was 6 or lower: $t(15) = 2.82$, $p < .05$.

Mastery variables appear in Table 4. Individuals with an Aspirational Ratio of 3.50 or higher made more attempts to solve the unsolvable puzzle task as compared with those with a W:M ratio of 1.89 or lower: $t(16) = 2.46$, $p < .05$. We also note a trend for those with W:M scores of 2.00–3.00 (medium group) to make more attempts than the low group: $t(13) = 2.11$, $p = .051$. Participants with a (high group) ZSum score greater than 40.00 reported higher levels of perceived agency as compared with those with a (medium group) ZSum score between 31.50 and 37.50: $t(15) = 2.94$, $p < .05$. The difference between the low and high ZSum groups approached significance: $t(14) = 1.70$, $p = .11$. We noted the slight curvilinear distribution of agency scores across the levels of ZSum. Consequently, we divided ZSum into two levels (low ZSum = 7.50–37.50; high ZSum = 40.00–88.00). The difference in Agency was statistically significant, low ZSum = 13.12 ($SD = 1.12$), high ZSum = 14.29 ($SD = .88$); $t(23) = 2.57$, $p < .05$; Cohen's d effect size =1.17.

Table 3. Construct validation of Rorschach hope variables: survival hope

Cognitive Triad Inventory			
		Resiliency Factor	
	N	M	SD
Raw D Score (resources – demands)[a]			
(−9.50−−.50) Low	9	11.00	2.64
(0–2.50) Medium	9	13.56	3.28
(3.50–17.00) High	7	15.29	3.04
Low vs. high: $t(14) = 3.01$, $p < .01$ (Cohen's d effect size = 1.51)			
Low vs. medium: $t(16) = 1.82$, $p = .08$ (Cohen's d effect size = .87)			
Ways of Coping Scale			
		Total Score	
	N	M	SD
Active + passive movement[b]			
(2.00–6.00) Low	10	15.21	1.43
(7.00–9.00) Medium	8	17.00	6.60
(10.00–19.00) High	7	19.14	4.44
Low vs. high $t(15) = 2.82$, $p < .05$ (Cohen's d effect size = 1.33)			

Note. [a]Derived mean of Exner (2003): Extratensives and introversives = .61 (raw D, EA – es). [b]Mean of Exner (2003): Extratensives and introversives = 9.87.

Retrospective Application of the Hope Index to a Case of Complete Suicide

In Table 5, we present the Rorschach Hope Index as applied to a documented case of suicide. The case summary is from *Rorschach Workshops* (Ritzler, 1998).

Law enforcement personnel admitted a 21-year-old man to a psychiatric facility. They found the young man trying to jump from a bridge. A reassessment occurred after 5 weeks. The battery included the Rorschach as well as the MMPI, a sentence completion test, and several projective drawings. The only data retained by Rorschach Workshops were the 13 MMPI T-Scores and the Rorschach responses. The MMPI validity scores were consistent with a *faking good* profile (higher L and K, lower F scales). The highest clinical scale score was Depression (71), followed by Hysteria (69) and Masculinity-Femininity (69), then Schizophrenia (66). The remaining clinical scales were within one standard deviation of the normative mean.

Four days after testing, the staff released him on a weekend pass, noting he appeared much improved. The patient then died by suicide after jumping from the same bridge.

Table 4. Construct validation of Rorschach hope variables: mastery hope

	Unsolvable Puzzle Task		
	Attempts (N)		
	N	M	SD
W:M (aspiration ratio)[a]			
(0.86–1.89) Low	10	3.50	0.85
(2.00–3.00) Medium	7	3.43	0.98
(3.50–8.00) High	8	4.88	2.10

Low vs. high: $t(16) = 2.46$, $p < .05$ (Cohen's d effect size = .94)
Medium vs. high: $t(13) = 2.11$, $p = .051$ (Cohen's d effect size = .94)

	Snyder Hope Scale		
	Agency subscale		
	N	M	SD
ZSum (exploratory drive)[b]			
(7.50–30.00) Low	8	13.39	1.19
(31.50–37.50) Medium	9	12.89	1.05
(40.00–88.00) High	8	14.28	0.88

Low vs. high: $t(14) = 1.70$, $p < .11$ (Cohen's d effect size = .86)
Medium vs. high: $t(15) = 2.94$, $p < .05$ (Cohen's d effect size = 1.44)

Note. [a]Mean of Exner (2003): Extratensives and introversives = 2.12. [b]Mean of Exner (2003): Extratensives and introversives = 38.

The individual had experienced a number of interpersonal challenges. He was born in the United States to immigrant parents. His father was an alcoholic who physically abused his mother. The mother had a history of serious mental illness that included psychotic, religiously toned delusions. When he was three, his parents separated. Other relatives assumed responsibility for his care. At college, he lived in a minority-segregated fraternity. He always felt uncomfortable in interpersonal situations, had few friends, and felt unliked. He was of above average intelligence and in good academic standing.

The following key elements of the Structural Summary are provided: $R = 22$; Lambda = 1.20; Control and Stress Tolerance, $EA = 4.5$, $es = 5$; Ideation, Ma: Mp = 3: 0; Mediation, $X+\% = .50$; Affect, $Afr = .38$; Processing, W: M = 8: 3, Interpersonal Perception, COP = 0; Self Perception, Egocentricity Index = .32. This individual's protocol was positive for just four of seven indicators on the (DEPI) Depression Index (57%) and only three of 12 indicators on the (SCON) Suicide Constellation (25%). In effect, his Rorschach protocol was negative for both depression and suicidal risk. (The clinical thresholds are five for DEPI and eight for SCON.)

Table 5. Case example: Application of the Hope Index to an undetected death by suicide

Rorschach Hope variable	Sample[a]	Exner (2003)[b]	Cutoff[c]	Death by suicide
Attachment hope				
Good human representation (GHR)	5.48	5.31	< 5.00	3 (below)
Cooperative movement (COP)	2.07	2.14	< 2.00	0 (below)
Survival hope				
Raw D (resources − demands)	0.75	0.61	< 0	−0.5 (below)
Active + passive movement	8.30	9.87	< 8.00	6 (below)
Mastery hope				
Aspirational ratio (W:M)	3.01	2.12	< 2.00	2.67 (above)
Exploratory drive (ZSum)[d]	36	38	< 36	36 (border)

Note. [a]Present research sample. [b]Exner (2003) norms are means of extratensives and introversives. [c]Proposed cutoffs for low hope. [d]ZSum norm derived from Zf and Zes tables.

Instructors feature this case in Rorschach training workshops as it represents a frustrating example of a false negative. A key to understanding the failed prediction is the presence of a high Lambda, indicative of possible avoidance and suggestive of a protocol that may be lacking in transparency. (This finding is cross-validated by the MMPI validity scale pattern.) Access to the original protocol makes it possible to compute a Hope Index. Despite a high Lambda, the derived Rorschach hope score creates an ominous clinical picture. Using cutoffs derived from the present research as well as Exner's (2003) norms, the protocol receives a score of 2 (maximum = 6). The individual fell below the cutoff on four of the six hope elements (67%).

Discussion

We validated six Rorschach variables against standard measures of three defining elements of hope: attachment, coping–survival, and mastery. To assess discriminant validity, we attempted a cross-comparison of each Rorschach variable with the other validation measure in each cluster (attachment through mastery). For example, we paired GHR with Self–Other Balance, Sum of A:P Movements with Resiliency, and W:M with Agency. We did not find any significant relationships (all $p > .05$). This suggests we are tapping unique dimensions of hope with the proposed six Rorschach variables. In the realm of attachment, GHR appear to reflect (emotional) trust while the perception of Cooperative Movement may relate to hope-derived action tendencies (connection and collaboration).

Nevertheless, in the course of human development, motives will invariably cross-fertilize. Early attachments influence survival and mastery patterns. Survival-related events such as loss or illness can affect attachment and mastery behaviors. For example, when scoring a variable such as Cooperative Movement, we are probably capturing elements of the survival and mastery system as well as attachment. There are two ways we can approach this issue. Investigators can launch further studies aiming to better untangle Rorschach derivatives of the motive systems underlying hope. Alternatively, we may arrive at an agreed-upon set of Rorschach variables that suffice to capture a blend of attachment, survival, and mastery aspects inextricably bound by development.

As predicted, Raw *D*, a measure of available psychic resources, related to a measure of perceived resiliency, and a greater number of Active and Passive Movement Responses were associated with more ways of coping. One might view these two dimensions of hope-based survival in terms of depth versus breadth of adaptation. Classic metaphors of hope include both a form of light (vital energy) and a network of bridges (coping strategies). Two of the oldest definitions of hope are an island in the middle of a wasteland and the notion of hopping from place to place (Simpson & Weiner, 1989).

Individuals with higher W:M scores demonstrated greater persistence on an unsolvable puzzle task. Those with higher *Z*Sum scores reported a stronger sense of personal agency for achieving goals. One interpretation is that the former (W:M) relates to prereflective, immediate goal engagement behavior (effort or persistence) while the latter (*Z*Sum) is more predictive of a reflective and summative goal-related attitude. We note that the Snyder Agency Scale includes items such as, "I have been pretty successful in life," "I meet the goals that I set for myself," and "My past experiences have prepared me well for my future." Kohut's (1971) distinction between ambition and ideals is possibly relevant in this context. While the W:M variable may address ambition, the *Z*Sum variable might correlate with perceptions of the idealized self as an agent who does not overlook environmental cues for goals advancement.

Correspondence Among the Hope Index, DEPI, and SCON

The Hope Index (total score, 0–6) showed little overlap with either the Exner Depression Index (DEPI, 0–7) or the Exner Suicide Constellation (SCON, 0–12). In both cases, the degree of shared variance was less than 3%. The Hope Index includes attachment, mastery, and survival hope. By contrast, only one of the seven DEPI variables and two of the 12 SCON variables deal with interpersonal resources. The DEPI does not contain any markers for coping or goal attainment. The SCON has one coping marker (EA > es) and one goal/achievement marker

(Zd). Both of the DEPI and SCON place the greatest weight on the presence of internal psychic pain (6/7 markers for DEPI and 6/12 for SCON). It is clear that depressive and suicidal states involve intense subjective distress. However, prolonged bouts of goal frustration, alienation, and perceived entrapment can also engender profound states of despair and desperation. Moreover, in the case of suicide, the clinical literature points to the ephemeral nature of a subjective state that is intermittent, waxing and waning (Bolton, 2015; Exner, 2003; Hawgood & De Leo, 2016). In short, placing too much emphasis on psychic pain in the assessment of depression and suicide not only ignores other critical dimensions of hope, but places the diagnostician in the difficult role of trying to capture a fleeting window of turmoil that is alternately coalescing and dissolving, sometimes in a matter of days, if not hours.

Revisiting the Case of Death by Suicide

We revisit the case of death by suicide presented earlier. Putting aside for a moment the young man's low hope score, one strength that emerged is a slightly above average Aspirational Ratio, not surprising for someone with a history of academic success and above average intelligence. He also achieved the minimal suggested ZSum score of 36, possibly the result of a lifelong attempt to integrate multiple dimensions of identity including sexuality, race, achievement, and community. His lack of Cooperative Movement and GHR aligns with the social isolation documented in his case history. His Raw *D* score was low, suggesting reduced flexibility as well as a limited depth of coping resources. He had twice as many Active Movement responses (4) as Passive Movement responses (2). However, consistent with our contention that the combination of Active and Passive Movement responses may be more important in the assessment of hope, his combined sum of six was 40% lower than the group average of those who scored higher in these ways of coping.

The picture emerges of an individual who may demonstrate a strong work ethic (W:M) and some ability to integrate the diversity within and around him (ZSum). He does not have a very positive view of others and is low in trust (GHR and COP). His coping profile reflects low stress tolerance (Raw *D*) and a reduced repertoire of coping strategies (Active and Passive Movement). His status as a good student probably lent an element of strength that masked his other hope deficits, particularly in the interpersonal and coping domains. The fact that mastery resources alone were not sufficient to sustain this young man begs a larger question. Is it time for psychology and psychiatry to re-evaluate the longstanding tradition of placing goal estimations at the center of their approaches to hope? (See also commentaries in Larsen & Stege, 2012; Scioli et al., 2011.)

Implications for Assessment and Future Research

This study is part of a larger research program to present hope in its full complexity. The findings as well as the case review reinforce a multidimensional view of hope in terms of attachment, survival/coping resources, and mastery. To illustrate the need for a fuller conceptualization of hope, we compared scores on the Hope Index with results on the Beck Hopelessness Scale (BHS), given to the study participants as a secondary assessment. The correlation between the Hope Index and BHS score was minimal ($r = .13$, $p > .05$), suggesting a shared variance of less than 2%. We computed a separate set of correlations for each of the three elements of the Hope Index and the BHS. Not surprisingly, the largest correlation involved Mastery ($r = .20$) with the other two dimensions of hope approaching a zero correlation (Rorschach Hope Index Attachment and BHS: $r = -.01$; Hope Index Survival and BHS: $r = .08$). All p values were $> .05$.

Investigators may wish to explore whether there are other Rorschach variables to address the hope elements of attachment, survival, or mastery (e.g., other aspects of organizational activity or stimulus engagement along with additional indicators of interpersonal perception or coping resources). In conducting such inquiries, it will be important to keep in mind the nature of hope (empowerment and goal orientation; trust, openness, and connectedness; self-regulation and perceived liberation). At some point, spirituality should factor into the Rorschach hope assessment process. It may be necessary to adopt a modified Rorschach procedure to capture this dimension of hope. One possible solution would be to insert another association phase after the first round of exposure to the cards, and before the inquiry phase. The examiner might prompt the individual with the following instructions: "Some individuals see religious or spiritual symbols when looking at these cards. Let's go through them a second time and see if you notice any religious or spiritual symbols or objects." We believe that spirituality functions to reinforce the underlying needs served by hope. With this in mind, a scoring algorithm for spirituality might include counts of good or bad responses related to spiritual presence or alienation (attachment), coping support or threat (survival), empowerment or repudiation (mastery). Research may reveal whether all 10 cards are necessary for eliciting religious or spiritual associations or if a selected subset will suffice.

One test case is inadequate for assessing the predictive validity of a new assessment tool. Retrospective studies of cases involving attempted suicides or death by suicide may be valuable but there will ultimately be a need for prospective studies. These investigations will yield firmer cutoff levels to aid in discriminating levels of hopelessness and degrees of risk.

Clinicians often focus on three variables when gauging suicidal risk: suicidal ideation, depression, and hopelessness (e.g., Osman et al., 2005; Posner et al., 2011). The introduction of multiple criteria begs the question of relative importance. One possible approach is to divide the window of concern into long, intermediate, and short-term timeframes. Assessment of depression appears most relevant when taking a long view whereas suicidal ideation is most critical to evaluate in the short term. The critical time in between may involve the development of increasing levels of hopelessness.

To capture a rising tide of despair, risk assessment protocols might include a battery of implicit and explicit measures that encompass three, if not four, of the hope dimensions (attachment through spirituality).

Beyond Suicide Assessment: Other Potential Uses of the Hope Index

The value of a robust measure of hope is not limited to predicting suicidal risk. Practitioners interested in the welfare of at-risk youth, vulnerable elders, the addicted, and others with various forms of debilitating mental illness cannot ignore levels of hope and despair. Health-care professionals who tend to individuals with a life-threatening physical illness and must convince them to endure painful medical regimen and risky interventions without guarantee of success must also be cognizant of waning hope.

A multidimensional hope assessment yields a profile of strengths and weakness. For example, the individual who ended his life clearly demonstrated a weakness in the social and coping domains. For another individual, the deficit may lie in the realm of goal engagement. With further research, it may be possible to generate specific treatment recommendations based on a Rorschach hope profile.

Several other methodological issues remain. There is a need for additional research comparing self-report inventories and external behavioral signs with the Hope Index as well as other potential methods of assessing hope (e.g., IAT or TAT methods). Are certain elements of hope (e.g., attachment or spirituality) more or less amenable to particular assessment strategies? Currently the Exner Suicide Constellation is invalid for individuals younger than 14 years. Future studies might address whether the Hope Index is valid for younger individuals. Will a [Youth] Hope Index require a modification of cutoffs, or substantial changes to incorporate developmental shifts in the structure of hope?

Acknowledgments

The authors wish to acknowledge the input and suggestions of the late John Exner Jr. and several anonymous reviewers, in the evolution of this manuscript.

References

Abramson, L. Y., Metalsky, G. I., & Alloy, L. B. (1989). Hopelessness depression: A theory-based subtype of depression. *Psychological Review, 96*(2), 358–372.

Anderson, K. W., & Skidmore, J. R. (1995). Empirical analysis of factors in depressive cognition: The Cognitive Triad Inventory. *Journal of Clinical Psychology, 51*(5), 603–609. https://doi.org/10.1002/1097-4679(199509)51:5<603::AID-JCLP2270510504>3.0.CO;2-Z

Beck, A. T. (1976). *Cognitive therapy and the emotional disorders*. New York, NY: International Universities Press.

Beck, A. T., Steer, R. A., & Brown, G. A. (1996). *BDI-II, Beck Depression Inventory: Manual*. San Antonio, TX: The Psychological Corporation.

Beck, A. T., Weissman, A., Lester, D., & Trexler, L. (1974). The measurement of pessimism: The Hopelessness Scale. *Journal of Consulting and Clinical Psychology, 42*(6), 861–865.

Beckham, E. E., Leber, W. R., Watkins, J. T., Boyer, J. L., & Cook, J. B. (1986). Development of an instrument to measure Beck's cognitive triad: The Cognitive Triad Inventory. *Journal of Consulting and Clinical Psychology, 54*(4), 566–567.

Bloch, E. (1986). *The principle of hope* (Vol. 1), Cambridge, MA: MIT Press.

Bolton, J. M. (2015). Suicide risk assessment in the emergency department: Out of the darkness. *Depression and Anxiety, 32*(2), 73–75.

Breznitz, S. (1986). The effect of hope on coping with stress. In M. H. Appley & P. Trumbull (Eds.), *Dynamics of stress: Physiological, psychological and social perspectives* (pp. 295–307). New York, NY: Plenum.

Cohen, J. (1988). *Statistical power analysis for the behavioral sciences*. Hillsdale, NJ: Lawrence Erlbaum.

Coughlan, K., Tata, P., & MacLeod, A. K. (2017). Personal goals, well-being and deliberate self-harm. *Cognitive Therapy and Research, 41*(3), 434–443.

Czopp, S., & Zeligman, R. (2016). The Rorschach Comprehensive System (CS) psychometric validity of individual variables. *Journal of Personality Assessment, 98*(4), 335–342.

DeGroot, K., Boeke, S., Bonke, B., & Passchier, J. (1997). A reevaluation of the adaptiveness of avoidant and vigilant coping with surgery. *Psychology and Health, 12*(5), 711–717.

Dufault, K., & Martocchio, B. (1985). Hope: Its spheres and dimensions. *Nursing Clinics of North America, 20*(2), 379–391.

Durkheim, E. (1951/1897). *Suicide*. New York, NY: The Free Press. (Original work published 1897).

Erikson, E. H. (1950). *Childhood and society*. New York, NY: Norton.

Exner, J. E. (1992). A conceptual critique of the EA: es comparison in the Comprehensive Rorschach System: Comment. *Psychological Assessment, 4*(3), 297–300.

Exner, J. E. (2003). *The Rorschach: A comprehensive system. Vol. 1. Basic foundations and principles of interpretation* (4th ed.). New York, NY: Wiley.

Folkman, S. (2010). Stress, coping, and hope. *Psycho-Oncology, 19*(9), 901–908.

Folkman, S., & Lazarus, R. S. (1985). If it changes it must be a process: Study of emotion and coping during three stages of a college examination. *Journal of Personality & Social Psychology, 48*(1), 150–170.

Forintos, D. P., Rózsa, S., Pilling, J., & Kopp, M. (2013). Proposal for a short version of the Beck Hopelessness Scale based on a national representative survey in Hungary. *Community Mental Health Journal, 49*(6), 822–830.

Frank, J. D. (1974). Psychotherapy: The restoration of morale. *The American Journal of Psychiatry, 131*(3), 271–274.

Franklin, J. C., Ribeiro, J. D., Fox, K. R., Bentley, K. H., Kleiman, E. M., Huang, X., & Nock, M. K. (2017). Risk factors for suicidal thoughts and behaviors: A meta-analysis of 50 years of research. *Psychological Bulletin, 143*(2), 187–232.

Glass, D. L., & Singer, J. E. (1972). *Urban stress*. New York, NY: Academic Press.

Godfrey, J. J. (1987). *A philosophy of human hope*. Dordrecht, The Netherlands: Martinus Nijhoff.

Gottschalk, L. A. (1985). Hope and other deterrents to illness. *American Journal of Psychotherapy, 39*(4), 515–525.

Hadley, S. A., & MacLeod, A. K. (2010). Conditional goal-setting, personal goals and hopelessness about the future. *Cognition and Emotion, 24*(7), 1191–1198.

Hagan, C. R., Podlogar, M. C., Chu, C., & Joiner, T. E. (2015). Testing the interpersonal theory of suicide: The moderating role of hopelessness. *International Journal of Cognitive Therapy, 8*(2), 99–113.

Hawgood, J., & De Leo, D. (2016). Suicide prediction – a shift in paradigm is needed. *Crisis, 37*(4), 251–255. https://doi.org/10.1027/0227-5910/a000440

Kohut, H. (1971). *The analysis of the self: A systematic approach to the psychoanalytic treatment of narcissistic personality disorders*. Chicago, IL: University of Chicago Press.

Kovacs, M., Beck, A. T., & Wiessman, A. (1975). Hopelessness: An indicator of suicidal risk. *Suicide, 5*, 98–103.

LaBarbera, J. D., & Cornsweet, C. (1985). Rorschach predictors of therapeutic outcome in a child psychiatric inpatient service. *Journal of Personality Assessment, 49*(2), 120–124.

Larsen, D. J., & Stege, R. (2012). Client accounts of hope in early counseling sessions: A qualitative study. *Journal of Counseling & Development, 90*(1), 45–54.

Lester, A. (1995). *Hope in pastoral care and counseling*. Louisville, KY: Westminster John Knox Press.

Lynch, W. F. (1965). *Images of hope: Imagination as healer of the hopeless*. Baltimore, MD: Helicon Press.

Marcel, G. (1962/1944). Homo Viator: Introduction to a metaphysic of hope. New York, NY: Harper and Row. (Original work published 1944).

Menninger, K. (1959). The academic lecture: Hope. *The American Journal of Psychiatry, 116*, 481–491.

Mihura, J. L., Meyer, G. J., Dumitrascu, N., & Bombel, G. (2013). The validity of individual Rorschach variables: Systematic reviews and meta-analyses of the comprehensive system. *Psychological Bulletin, 139*(3), 548–605.

Mowrer, O. H. (1960). *Learning theory and behavior*. New York, NY: Wiley.

Nowotny, M. (1989). Assessment of hope in patients with cancer: Development of an instrument. *Oncology Nursing Forum, 16*(1), 57–61.

Osman, A., Gutierrez, P. M., Barrios, F. X., Bagge, C. L., Kopper, B. A., & Linden, S. (2005). The Inventory of Suicide Orientation-30: Further validation with adolescent psychiatric inpatients. *Journal of Clinical Psychology, 61*(4), 481–497.

Posner, K., Brown, G. K., Stanley, B., Brent, D. A., Yershova, K. V., & Oquendo, M. A., . . . Mann, J. J. (2011). The Columbia-Suicide Severity Rating Scale: Initial validity and internal consistency findings from three multisite studies with adolescents and adults. *The American Journal of Psychiatry, 168*(12), 1266–1277. https://doi.org/10.1176/appi.ajp.2011.10111704

Pruyser, P. W. (1987). Maintaining hope in adversity. *Bulletin of the Menninger Clinic, 5*(51), 463–474.

Rand, K. L. (2009). Hope and optimism: Latent structures and influences on grade expectancy and academic performance. *Journal of Personality, 77*(1), 231–260.

Ritzler, B. (1998, Spring). *Rorschach scoring and interpretation*. Rorschach Workshops, Asheville, NC.
Rosen, G. (1971). History in the study of suicide. *Psychological Medicine, 1*(4), 267–285.
Rothbaum, F., Weisz, J. R., & Snyder, S. S. (1982). Changing the world and changing the self: A two-process model of perceived control. *Journal of Personality and Social Psychology, 42*(1), 5–37.
Rotter, J. B. (1967). A new scale for the measurement of interpersonal trust. *Journal of Personality, 35*(4), 651–665.
Scioli, A., & Biller, H. B. (2009). *Hope in the age of anxiety*. New York, NY: Oxford University Press.
Scioli, A., MacNeil, S., Partridge, V., Tinker, E., & Hawkins, E. (2012). Hope, HIV and health: A prospective study. *AIDS Care, 24*(2), 149–156.
Scioli, A., Ricci, M., Nyugen, T., & Scioli, E. R. (2011). Hope: Its nature and measurement. *Psychology of Religion and Spirituality, 3*(2), 78–97.
Scioli, A., Scioli-Salter, E. R., Sykes, K., Anderson, C., & Fedele, M. (2016). The positive contributions of hope to maintaining and restoring health: An integrative, mixed-method approach. *The Journal of Positive Psychology, 11*(2), 135–148.
Simpson, J., & Weiner, E. (1989). *The Oxford English dictionary*. Northamptonshire, UK: Oxford University Press.
Snyder, C. R., Harris, C., Anderson, J. R., Holleran, S. A., Irving, L. M., & Sigmon, S. T. Harney, P. (1991). The will and ways: Development and validation of an individual-differences measure of hope. *Journal of Personality and Social Psychology, 60*(4), 570–585.
Stotland, E. (1969). *The psychology of hope*. San Francisco, CA: Jossey-Bass.
White, R. W. (1959). Motivation reconsidered: The concept of competence. *Psychological Review, 66*(5), 297–333.
Wright, B. A., & Shontz, F. (1968). Process and tasks in hoping. *Rehabilitation Literature, 29*(11), 322–331.
Wright, T. L., & Tedeschi, R. G. (1975). Factor analysis of the Interpersonal Trust Scale. *Journal of Consulting and Clinical Psychology, 43*(4), 470–477.

Received October 9, 2015
Revision received June 6, 2018
Accepted August 10, 2018
Published online November 9, 2018

Anthony Scioli
Department of Psychology
Keene State College
Keene, NH 03431
USA
tscioli@keene.edu

Summary

In this study, we derived a measure of hope from the Rorschach. Drawing on an integrative approach to hope (Scioli et al., 2011), we identified six Rorschach variables representing two dimensions each of the following: interpersonal perceptions, coping resources, or goal engagement. These variables are GHR, COP, Raw D, Active and Passive Movement, the Aspiration Index, and ZSum. We conducted an empirical study of 25 young adults, tested individually with the Rorschach and standard questionnaires as well as a classic puzzle task (possible and impossible). For purposes of validation, we divided each Rorschach variable into three groups of low, medium, and high. The one exception was COP (low or high, 0 or 1+). The group cutoff values followed an analysis of sample frequency distributions as well as existing norms (Exner, 2003). We validated each variable against theoretically linked measures of attachment, stress tolerance, and mastery. In five analyses, significant differences emerged between low and high levels of a Rorschach variable. In four other analyses, the significant differences were between low and medium groups or medium and high groups. At least one significant group difference emerged for each Rorschach variable (Cohen's d = .86–1.51). There was little overlap between the Hope Index and either the SCON (2.9% shared variance) or the DEPI (3.2%).

We propose a Rorschach State Hope Index and tentative cutoff values for each variable (single variable: scored 0 or 1; total score range: 0–6). We applied the Hope Index retrospectively to a college student who completed suicide despite a relatively low scores on both the Suicide Constellation and the DEPI. The young man was of above average intelligence and academically strong. He had few friends and felt uncomfortable in social situations. He fell below the cutoff on four of the six Hope Index variables (GHR and COP [Attachment]; Raw D and Active: Passive Movement [Coping]). His aspirational ratio fell below our sample mean but exceeded Exner (2003) norms, while his ZSum equaled our sample mean but fell below the Exner (2003) norms. This case illustrates the need for a multidimensional approach to hope theory and assessment, beyond the focus on goals and agency, which has dominated psychology and psychiatry. We conclude by suggesting other potential applications of a Rorschach Hope Index (e.g., health psychology and behavioral medicine).

Résumé

Dans cette étude, nous avons déduit une mesure de l'espoir à partir du test de Rorschach. En se fondant sur une approche intégrative de l'espoir (Scioli et coll. 2011), nous avons identifié six variables de Rorschach ; représentant chacune deux des dimensions suivantes : les perceptions interpersonnelles, les ressources d'adaptation ou l'engagement envers les objectifs. Les voici : GHR, COP, Score D, Mouvement actif et passif, l'Indice d'aspiration et ZSomme. Nous avons mené une étude empirique auprès de 25 jeunes adultes, testés individuellement avec le test de Rorschach et des questionnaires standards, ainsi qu'un casse-tête classique à résoudre (possible et impossible). Aux fins de validation, nous avons divisé chaque variable de Rorschach en trois groupes (faible, moyen et élevé), avec la variable COP pour seule exception (faible ou élevé, 0 ou 1+). Les valeurs seuils du groupe ont suivi une analyse des distributions de fréquence d'échantillonnage, ainsi que des normes existantes (Exner, 2003). Nous avons validé chaque variable par comparaison avec des mesures théoriquement corrélées de l'attachement, de la tolérance au stress et de la maîtrise. Dans cinq analyses, des différences significatives sont apparues entre les niveaux faible et élevé d'une même variable de Rorschach. Dans quatre autres analyses, les différences significatives ont concerné les groupes faible et moyen ou moyen et élevé. Nous avons constaté au moins une différence significative entre les groupes pour chaque variable de Rorschach (d de Cohen = 0,86 à 1,51). Le chevauchem6ent entre l'Indice d'espoir de Rorschach et la SCON (variance partagée de 2,9 %) ou le DEPI (3,2 %) était faible.

Nous proposons un Indice de l'état d'espoir de Rorschach et des valeurs seuils provisoires pour chaque variable (variable unique : score 0 ou 1 ; fourchette de score total : 0 à 6). Nous avons appliqué l'Indice d'espoir a posteriori à un étudiant universitaire qui s'est suicidé malgré un score relativement faible à la fois pour la Constellation Suicide et le DEPI (indice de dépression). Le jeune homme possédait une intelligence supérieure à la moyenne et obtenait de bons résultats scolaires. Il avait peu d'amis et se sentait mal à l'aise en société. Pour quatre des six variables de l'Indice d'espoir, ses résultats se sont révélés inférieurs aux valeurs seuils (GHR et COP [attachement] ; Score D et Mouvement actif/passif [adaptation]). Son Indice d'aspiration est tombé sous la moyenne de notre échantillon, mais a dépassé les normes Exner (2003), tandis que sa ZSomme a égalé à la moyenne de notre échantillon, mais s'est retrouvée inférieure aux normes Exner (2003). Ce cas illustre la nécessité d'une approche multidimensionnelle de la théorie et de l'évaluation de l'espoir. Nous devons en effet arrêter de nous focaliser uniquement sur les objectifs et le pouvoir d'action, comme cela a toujours prévalu dans les domaines de la psychologie et de la psychiatrie. En conclusion, nous suggérons de nouvelles applications potentielles associées à un Indice d'espoir de Rorschach (p. ex. en psychologie de la santé et en médecine comportementale).

要約

ロールシャッハHope指標の作成に向けて

本研究で我々は、ロールシャッハにおけるHope尺度を導き出した。

hopeに対する統合的アプローチ（Scioli et al., 2011）を用いながら、我々は、対人知覚と対処能力または ゴール設定の2つの特徴を表す6つのロールシャッハ変数を特定した。これらの変数は、GHR、COP、Dスコア、運動反応に伴うActiveとPassive、aspiration指数とZSumである。我々は、25人の青年に対して実証的な研究を行った。すなわちそれは、彼らにロールシャッハテスト、標準化された質問紙、そして古典的なパズル課題を個別に行った。検証のために、我々は、ロールシャッハの各変数について、低群・中群・高群の3つのグループに分けた。COPだけは例外的に、低群と高群または、0か1に分けられた。各グループのカットオフ値は、Exner (2003) のノーマルデータをサンプルとした度数分布により定めた。我々は、愛着、ストレス耐性および統制（原語；mastery）に理論上リンクする尺度に対してそれぞれの変数を検証した。5つの解析において、1つのロールシャッハ変数の低群と高群の間で有意差が認められた。他の4つの解析では低群と中群、中群と高群の間で有意差が認められた。各ロールシャッハ変数には、少なくとも1つの群に有意差が認められた（Cohen's d =.86-1.51）。Hope指数とSCON（2.9%の寄与率）、Hope指数とDEPI（3.2%）では、オーバーラップはほとんどなかった。

我々は、ロールシャッハHope指標とそれぞれの変数における仮のカットオフ値を提唱する（個別変数：0または1；総スコア範囲：0-6）。我々は、後ろ向きスタディにより、SCONとDEPIの両方において相対的に低値を示したにも関わらず、自殺をした一大学生にHope指標を適用した。その若者は、知能と学歴において平均以上であった。彼は、友達が少なく、社会的状況において不快感を持っていた。彼は、6つのHope指標変数（GHRとCOP〔愛着〕；DスコアとActive : Passive〔コーピング〕）のうち、4つでカットオフ値を下回っていた。彼のaspirational 比は、Exner (2003)標準を超えてはいたものの、我々のサンプルの平均を下回っていた。一方、彼のZSum 指標は、Exner (2003) 標準を下回っていたが、我々のサンプル平均と同等であった。

このケースは、心理学と精神医学に対して、hope理論とアセスメントの多元的アプローチの必要性を浮き彫りにしている。我々は、1つのロールシャッハHope指数を他の潜在的な適用、例えば健康心理学や行動心理学への適用を示唆しつつ本研究を結論づける。

Original Article

A Scientific Critique of Rorschach Research

Revisiting Exner's *Issues and Methods in Rorschach Research* (1995)

Jason M. Smith[1], Carl B. Gacono[2], Patrick Fontan[3], Enna E. Taylor[4], Ted B. Cunliffe[5], and Anne Andronikof[6]

[1]FCC Hazelton, Bruceton Mills, WV, USA
[2]Private Practice, Asheville, NC, USA
[3]Circonscription Saint Denis 1, Paris, France
[4]Private Practice, San Francisco, CA, USA
[5]Private Practice, Miami, FL, USA
[6]Laboratoire IPSé, Université Paris Ouest, Nanterre, France

Abstract: Exner's (1995a) *Issues and Methods in Rorschach Research* provided a standard of care for conducting Rorschach research; however, the extent to which studies have followed these guidelines has not been examined. Similarly, meta-analytic approaches have been used to comment on the validity of Exner's Comprehensive System (CS) variables without an evaluation as to the extent that individual studies have conformed to the proposed methodological criteria (Exner, 1995a; Gacono, Loving, & Bodholdt, 2001). In this article, 210 studies cited in recent meta-analyses by Mihura, Meyer, Dumitrascu, and Bombel (2013) were examined. The studies were analyzed in terms of being research on the Rorschach versus research with the Rorschach and whether they met the threshold of validity/generalizability related to specific Rorschach criteria. Only 104 of the 210 (49.5%) studies were research on the Rorschach and none met all five Rorschach criteria assessed. Trends and the need for more stringent methods when conducting Rorschach research were presented.

Keywords: Rorschach, Exner Comprehensive System, psychological assessment

Exner's (1995a) *Issues and Methods in Rorschach Research* set a standard of care for conducting Rorschach research. At that time, he stated: "A huge number of published investigations ... are clearly marked by errors in design, implementation, and/or analysis" (Exner, 1995b, p. 3). Since Exner's (1995a) cautions, no one has examined the degree to which Rorschach research has conformed to the guidelines offered by the chapter authors. Meta-analytic findings, in particular, have been accepted at face value with little consideration for the degree to which individual studies fell within the parameters outlined by Exner (1995a) and others (e.g., Gacono, Loving, & Bodholdt, 2001).

The following is a brief overview of each chapter in *Issues and Methods in Rorschach Research*. In addition to highlighting issues to be considered when conducting Rorschach research, Exner (1995b) cautioned the researcher to be aware of the complexity involved with this type of research. He presented many essential ideas such as: (1) offering cautions about small sample size (at least 15 subjects are needed in an experimental group for every dependent variable to be included in the analysis); (2) presenting considerations related to personality/response style (Lambda & Introversive/Extratensive); (3) suggesting how normative data can be misused (any comparisons with normative data would find meaningless significant results; "ingenuous conclusion that they have made a great discovery," p. 17); (4) cautioning against overemphasizing or overgeneralizing results; and (5) not using the "shotgun study" (p. 14) where there is no a priori model specified before analyzing Rorschach data. This latter approach can increase the probability of finding significant results by chance (Type I error; also see Viglione, 1995; Weiner, 1995b). Further, and most importantly, Exner stressed that not everything "appearing in the literature was truth" (p. 4).

Dies (1995a, 1995b) discussed issues with sample size (a sample size of less than 20 could lead to deceptive results due to deviant subjects), missing/inappropriate control groups, and problems related to administration/scoring (also see Exner, Kinder, & Curtis, 1995; Gacono, Evans, & Viglione, 2008; Ritzler & Exner, 1995). Dies also opined that a theoretical model needs to proceed a study and it guides analyses (also Weiner, 1995b). Likewise, he identified certain Rorschach studies that had methodological bias, some of which were included in recent meta-analyses (e.g., Ball, Archer, Gordon, & French, 1991). Additionally, Dies (also see Acklin & McDowell, 1995; Mcguire, Kinder, Curtiss, & Viglione, 1995) found that researchers did not provide basic demographic data. This is necessary for interpreting findings, especially when a study is focused on validating the corollaries of a Rorschach variable, including sample parameters such as Lambda, Responses, mean, standard deviations, and frequencies for the variables studied (also see Gacono et al., 2001; Gacono & Gacono, 2008).

Viglione and Exner (1995) cautioned against inappropriate control groups (i.e., using an Exner normative sample as the comparison group; also see Shaffer, Erdberg, & Haroian, 1999 for other normative data) and stressed the importance of critically evaluating previous Rorschach literature. Failure to critique the literature can and has allowed studies with inaccurate and ambiguous results to infiltrate published studies creating deceptive impressions (also see Cunliffe et al., 2012). Proper statistical methods were also discussed, specifically the importance of accurately applying parametric versus nonparametric statistical procedures (many Rorschach variables form J-shaped curves that are not conducive to analysis with parametric procedures; Viglione, 1995). Further, Viglione (1995) identified the variables appropriate for parametric and nonparametric statistics. Weiner (1995b) discussed the differences of using the Rorschach as a dependent and independent measure (doing research *with* the Rorschach or *on* the Rorschach), to provide adequate interrater reliabilities (80% agreement or better for Rorschach variables) and that poorly designed research will contain Type I and II error (stating a relationship exists when it does not or failing to identify relationships that exist). Ritzler and Exner (1995) discussed the limitations of clinical research and its chance for confounding variables (i.e., R, EB, and Lambda). Mcguire and colleagues (1995) stated that Rorschach variables may need to be categorized (i.e., dichotomous variables). Finally, Zillmer and Vuz (1995) provided information to perform factor analyses with Rorschach data.

Overall, many of the authors of *Issues and Methods in Rorschach Research* stressed the importance of not using a small sample size, providing key variables means/standard deviations (R, Lambda) as these can confound other variables, and the need to critically evaluate Rorschach research that may contain problems with methodology.

Gacono and colleagues (2001), Gacono and Gacono (2008), and Cunliffe et al. (2012) have added to the necessary parameters for conducting Rorschach research in order for a study to be generalizable and to allow reviewers to accurately interpret findings (e.g., reporting mean, standard deviation, and frequencies for IQ, Lambda, number of Responses). They offered five conceptual and four methodological criteria for evaluating the Rorschach/psychopathy research (Gacono et al., 2001, p. 32; also see Cunliffe et al., 2012; Gacono & Gacono, 2008; Gacono et al., 2008). Only Methodological Criteria 2–4 (see below) are provided as they apply to Rorschach research.

Methodological Issues in the Assessment of Rorschach/Psychopathy Findings (Gacono et al., 2001, p. 32)

2. Studies need to account for (control or delineate) the limitations imposed by factors such as gender, sexual deviance, concurrent Axis I psychosis, age, IQ, testing setting, and legal status. These factors can influence the production of certain Rorschach variables.
3. R (number of responses) must be considered. Increased R is found in certain sex offender groups, (Bridges, Wilson, & Gacono, 1998; Gacono, Meloy, & Bridges, 2000), whereas low R is typical among many criminal groups (Viglione, 1999). Thus, R can act as a moderator influencing the relationship

between Rorschach variables and criterion variables. Research should investigate this hypothesis by controlling for R and examining the relationship between Rorschach variables and criterion constructs at different levels of R (e.g., R = 14–17, etc.).
4. Response style must be considered (Bannatyne, Gacono, & Greene, 1999). Variables and styles such as R, Lambda, Extratensive, and Introversive can impact the production of certain Rorschach variables (Exner, 1995b), contributing to seemingly discrepant findings among studies.

While the wording of Methodological Criteria 2, 3, and 4 is geared toward Rorschach studies, similar issues (with modifications) are essential when conducting research with other psychological assessment instruments such as the Minnesota Multiphasic Personality Inventory-2 (MMPI-2; Butcher, Dahlstrom, Graham, Tellegen, & Kaemmer, 1989), Personality Assessment Inventory (PAI; Morey, 1991), or Millon Clinical Multiaxial Inventory – IV (MCMI-IV; Millon, Grossman, & Millon, 2015). These criteria (2, 3, and 4) will be expanded because they are important caveats for Rorschach research.

Potential confounds within the parameters of the instrument used should be assessed. Rorschach responses and protocol constriction can be significantly affected by mental illness, IQ, legal status, age, and testing environment (Methodological Criterion 2; Exner, 1974, 2003; Weiner, 1966). IQ and/or Educational level affect the production of certain research variables and must be accounted for by researchers (Exner, 2003; Gacono et al., 2001; Weiner, 1966). Meyer, Giromini, Viglione, Reese, and Mihura (2015) found years of adult education was correlated with different Rorschach variables related to complexity and cognitive synthesis. Therefore, a lack of consideration of these factors may result in methodological bias. Demographic information must be provided in order for reviewers to understand the meaning of any Rorschach data offered within the study.

As stated in Methodological Criterion 3, the number of Rorschach responses (R) relates to the stability and reliability of Rorschach variables (Viglione & Meyer, 2008; Weiner, 2003); protocols with less than 14 responses (R < 14) should be interpreted with caution as they typically do not have enough data for adequate retest reliability (Weiner, 2003). Although it is acknowledged that R < 14 protocols were considered acceptable if accompanied by a Lambda below 1.2 (Exner, 1986) and these protocols may have clinical significance (Gacono, 1997), the current standard per the Exner Comprehensive System (CS; Exner, 1993, 2003) requires 14 or more responses for interpretation. Further, the problem of R (Exner, 1992; Meyer, 1992; Wood, Nezworski, & Stejskal, 1996) may or may not impact Rorschach results; however, significant differences between experimental groups on R could impact research findings (Weiner, 1995a). One can state with greater certainty that within a Rorschach protocol of over 30 responses having a T or Fr + rF equal to zero, the absence of these variables was most likely due to either the absence of the trait or the personality functioning of the subject. In a protocol with less than 14 responses, additional hypotheses need to be considered. Similarly, in a protocol with 12 responses and four reflections it is highly likely that the presence of reflections are stating something about the personality of the person (Gacono & Meloy, 1994).

Methodological Criterion 4 includes participants with Lambda > .99 and/or F% = .50 (Meyer, Viglione, & Exner, 2001). These "response style variables" (Gacono & Gacono, 2008 –Lambda and R) are essential to interpreting Rorschach findings and are the two main validity criteria of a CS protocol (Exner, 2003). Further, if attempting to validate the Rorschach with meta-analyses, valid protocols (R and Lambda reported; R ≥ 14) are needed. Frequently seemingly discrepant findings can be explained by a predominance of high Lambda protocols in their samples (Exner provided different normative samples for Introversive/Extratensive patients for L > 0.99 & L < 1.00). Further, Konishi (2003) found differences in many Rorschach variables between high and low Lambda groups. While the "constriction" of the protocols is frequently interpretable related to the sample characteristics, comparing Rorschach variables between other studies (more normatively distributed Lambdas) is impossible (Gacono & Gacono, 2008). It would be difficult to know if the presence or absence of a CS variable is due to a high Lambda or the absence of the trait in a high Lambda sample. For example, if a study of male offenders had an overall mean L > .99 (high Lambda) and did not produce any reflections, it would be difficult to determine whether the lack of these variables was due to the protocol's constriction or the absence of the trait represented by these variables. Certainly, one cannot compare the high Lambda sample with a sample of male offenders with a mean L = .75 (avg. Lambda range) where these variables were present and then conclude that the negative findings in the high sample negate the positive findings in the more normally distributed sample. Assuming equality in the samples where one is a high Lambda sample is not justified. Generalizability is limited and only within-sample interpretive conclusions are justified. This reinforces the rationale for including Lambda means, standard deviations, etc. for all samples included in Rorschach research so the reviewer can determine whether the lack of results was due to this potential confound, which tends to create either a Type I (stating a relationship exists when it does not) or Type II error (failing to identify a relationship that does in fact exist).

As noted by Gacono and Gacono (2008) when discussing the validity versus generalizability of findings in their forensic outpatient groups:

Atypical patterns of constriction are common and frequently represent accurate portrayals of the patient's psychology (referring to high Lambda samples) ... For example, the higher rate of positive SCZI and PTI and Level 2 Special Scores among Schizophrenic groups...compared to our outpatient forensic groups does not indicate a lack of psychotic process among these patients. It also does not, necessarily, suggest resistance to the testing process. Rather, this finding must be interpreted in light of the patient's chronicity and their cognitive and emotional impoverishment. Rorschach constriction or expansion must always be explained within the context of the entire assessment battery and the patient's psychosocial history. (p. 443)

Researchers have also indicated the importance of determining and reporting interrater reliability for all Rorschach variables studied (Meyer, 1999; Viglione & Meyer, 2008; Weiner, 2003; Wood, Nezworski, & Stejskal, 1996). Therefore, researchers should report interrater reliability (≥ .60 [kappa and/or ICC] and 80% agreement is characterized as good to excellent; Meyer, 1999; Weiner, 1995a, 2003). Failure to report good/excellent interrater reliability is problematic as without reliability one is not assured of finding valid studies (Borsboom, Mellenbergh, & van Heerden, 2004).

Further, though there is no standard that is considered an adequate sample size; it appears that less than 20 is not acceptable using effect size, power, and alpha tables for nonparametric tests (Cohen, 1992; Dies, 1995a; Exner, 1995b). In neuroscience research, having small samples negatively impacts reliability and has less power (Button et al., 2013), and these points are also relevant for Rorschach research. Therefore, when a study has low statistical power there is less chance of detecting a true effect and "low power also reduces the likelihood that a statistically significant result reflects a true effect" (p. 365; Type II error). Low-sample research can also be viewed as unethical, inefficient, and wasteful (Button et al., 2013).

In summary, many different criteria need to be addressed when completing Rorschach research based on previous research from prominent Rorschach experts. However, five were selected that were mentioned most by many researchers and that appear to be essential for the validity and generalizability of research findings when conducting Rorschach research. These five are: (1) IQ/Educational level; (2) Rorschach Responses; (3) Lambda/F%; (4) interrater reliability; and (5) sample size.

These criteria are paramount for Rorschach research as there has been an increase in using meta-analyses with the Rorschach. Meta-analyses may overcome some of these problems such as small sample size, low power, and small effect sizes, unless the individual studies used in the meta-analyses contain problems related to these five criteria.

Meta-Analysis

Meta-analytic procedures are frequently utilized in assessing the validity of psychological measures (Sánchez-Meca & Marín-Martínez, 2010) including the Rorschach (Mihura et al., 2013; Wood et al., 2010). However, meta-analyses are only as good as the individual studies that they include (Button et al., 2013; Cunliffe et al., 2012; Hunter & Schmidt, 2004). For example, recent meta-analyses by Wood et al. (2010) examining the Rorschach and psychopathy were found to contain methodological bias in the research studies suggesting that there were not enough appropriate studies to perform the meta-analyses (see Cunliffe et al., 2012). Out of the 22 studies utilized in the meta-analyses, only one study was valid for inclusion by Rorschach/psychopathy standards (Cunliffe et al., 2012; Gacono et al., 2001; Gacono et al., 2008).

Recent meta-analyses by Mihura et al. (2013) questioned the validity of several Rorschach Comprehensive System (RCS; Exner, 2003) variables (e.g., Egocentricity Index and Isolation Index). Mihura et al. found mean validity coefficients of $r = .27$ when using the Rorschach variables against externally assessed criteria (e.g., psychiatric diagnosis) and $r = .08$ for introspectively assessed criteria (e.g., self-report measures). Further, effect sizes were calculated for the different Rorschach individual variables and they used Hemphill (2003) criteria to interpret the effect sizes. In total, 13 variables had excellent support (e.g., An + Xy; Perceptual Thinking Index; $r \geq .33$), 17 had good support (e.g., Lambda, Affective Ratio; $r \geq .21$), 10 had modest support (e.g., Vista, PHR; $r = .15-.21$), 13 had little or no support (e.g., Pure Color, Food; $r < .15$), and 12 variables (e.g., Aspiration Ratio, Color Projection) did not have any validity studies.

Wood, Garb, Nezworski, Lilienfeld, and Duke (2015) critiqued the Mihura et al. (2013) meta-analyses and indicated that the research by Mihura et al. was biased, since they failed to include certain articles/unpublished dissertations. Mihura, Meyer, Bombel, and Dumitrascu (2015) responded to these criticisms and refuted the claims of publication bias. Tibon Czopp and Zeligman (2016) also critiqued the Mihura et al. (2013) meta-analyses. Tibon Czopp and Zeligman focused their critique on the 13 CS variables that Mihura et al. stated had little to no support (e.g., Pure Color, Food; $r < .15$). They argued that these variables should not be removed from the CS system. They suggested there were discrepancies with the way Mihura and colleagues defined the 13 CS variables in the meta-analyses, which was not comparable to the customary CS interpretation for these variables. They argued the 13 individual variables needed to be interpreted within the CS clusters (e.g., self-perception, affective, etc.) due to the Rorschach being a multidimensional method. Additionally, in order to validate the 13 CS variables, externally assessed criteria (i.e., observer ratings, diagnosis) are better than introspectively assessed criteria (i.e., self-report measures). Tibon Czopp and Zeligman also postulated that there may have been studies on these 13 CS variables. These studies that were not included in the meta-analyses may have supported the CS variables. Therefore, findings that actually existed were not revealed in the Mihura et al. meta-analyses (Type II error). Mihura, Meyer, Bombel, and Dumitrascu (2016) responded, saying the statements used by Tibon Czopp and Zeligman were biased, their arguments would have lowered validity coefficients, and they needed to perform their own meta-analyses for these 13 variables.

There are different ways to critically evaluate studies within a meta-analysis. One way to evaluate validity (Borsboom et al., 2004), especially relevant to Rorschach studies, is to determine whether the articles used were studies *with the Rorschach* (application studies) or studies *on the Rorschach* (validation studies; Weiner, 1995b). Another way to conceptualize this would be using the Rorschach as the dependent variable (application) or the independent variable (validation). Typically, in application studies (studies with the Rorschach), Rorschach variables are assumed to be valid measures of a specific psychological construct and they can be replaced by another instrument measuring the same construct. A validation study would be attempting to determine the Rorschach variable meaning and it does not assume it is already valid. An example of an application study would be a researcher studying cognitive remediation effects on thought disorder in patients with schizophrenia. This researcher might choose to assess thought disorder with the Rorschach CS WSum6 variable. However, the WSum6 score could be replaced by the Thought and Language Disorder Scale (Kircher et al., 2014) without modification to the experimental design (thought disorder could be operationalized differently). In this example, the researcher assumes that the WSum6 score is already a valid measure of thought disorder. Although this example would seem to support concurrent validity of both psychological measures, the correlation may not be a true estimate of validity (Borsboom et al., 2004). Therefore, construct validity may be more important as without constructs and theory, psychology would not be classified as a science (Dies, 1995a). By nature, application studies (*with* the Rorschach) are not designed to validate specific Rorschach variables, rather they are used to study a clinical phenomenon. It would be problematic to use application studies (*with* the Rorschach) – which were not designed to *validate* Rorschach variables – in order to evaluate the *validity* of Rorschach scores. Ideally, meta-analyses on the validity of individual Rorschach variables should be based on validation studies (i.e., studies *on* the Rorschach; also see Borsboom et al., 2004).

Another method for assessing individual studies in a meta-analysis is to evaluate specific criteria relevant to the instrument or procedure studied (Cunliffe et al., 2012; Gacono et al., 2001). Hunter and Schmidt (2004) outlined the necessary components of a meta-analytic study: author, date, sample size, standardized effect score, subject characteristics, diagnostic conditions (scope, duration, and severity), strength of study design, and individual study methodological concerns. Validity forms the basis of Hunter and Schmidt's (2004) comments concerning the importance of ensuring that reliable, valid, and methodologically sound studies are selected for inclusion in a meta-analysis. Further, although researchers appear to use mathematically sound methods (equations used as intended), the issue lies in the validity (i.e., meaning; Borsboom et al., 2004) of the application of these techniques to methodologically biased studies included in a meta-analysis. Therefore, it is important to analyze the Rorschach studies included in a specific meta-analysis and to evaluate them with specific criteria (e.g., sample size, interrater reliability).

Present Study

In this article, the studies from the Mihura et al. (2013) meta-analyses were analyzed examining the quality of the study in light of Exner (1995a) and others (Cunliffe et al., 2012; Gacono et al., 2001). The 210 studies (similar to Dies, 1995b) from the Mihura et al. (2013) meta-analyses were examined focusing on whether the articles were application or validation studies (studies *with* the Rorschach vs. studies *on* the Rorschach) as well as the five methodological Rorschach criteria related to the validity and generalizability discussed by many Rorschach researchers. The five criteria were: (1) IQ/Education level; (2) Responses; (3) Lambda/F%; (4) interrater reliability; and (5) sample size.

Method

All articles used in the Mihura et al. (2013) meta-analyses were obtained and reviewed. Then, all 210 articles were examined for the following five main areas:
1. IQ/Education level,
2. Responses,
3. Lambda/F%,
4. Interrater reliability, and
5. Sample size.

Within each five criteria, different questions were examined. The issues were tallied up and a sum total for all 210 articles was obtained when the answer to the questions (see below) was *no*. Therefore, the examinations were:

1. IQ/Education level
   a. Did the article have statistics related to IQ/Educational level (*M* and range)?
   b. If either mean or range was provided, did the article include both statistics?
   c. If IQ range was reported, did all participants have an IQ > 80?

2. Responses (R)
   a. Did the article have statistics related to R (*M* and range)?
   b. If mean was provided, did the article include range?
   c. If range was provided, did the article include mean?
   d. If range was reported, did all protocols have R ≥ 14?

3. Lambda/F%
   a. Did the article have statistics related to Lambda/F% (*M* and range)?
   b. If mean was provided, were the means for Lambda/F% < 0.99/50%?
   d. If mean was provided, did the article report range?
   d. If the mean of Lambda/F% > .99/.50, did the article report IQ/Education Level? (L/F% > .99/.50 and IQ/Education level were examined in combination as this affects generalizability.)

4. Interrater reliability
   a. Did the article have interrater reliability statistics?
   b. If interrater reliability was reported, were there values for ICC/κ ≥ .60 or ≥ 80% agreement?

5. Sample size
   a. Did the article have comparison groups with ≥ 20 participants?

An overall analysis of the 210 articles was conducted after the aforementioned analyses. This was to determine how many problems an article had with the five main criteria. For example, if an article did not report Lambda and interrater reliability statistics, it was calculated that the study had two methodological issues. Therefore, the five criteria were tallied up to determine how many problems an article had (i.e., the article contained zero, one, two, etc. problems).

After assessing issues in the 210 articles, the articles were then classified as either validation or application studies. See the previous section to understand how validation and application studies were operationalized. After identifying the validation studies, and since they are preferred for meta-analyses, these articles were reviewed with the same five criteria as all 210 articles.

Due to the importance of validation studies in a meta-analysis, only these articles were examined to determine whether the methodological bias stated earlier had an impact on findings. The validation studies were reviewed to determine whether there were any counterintuitive findings. A counterintuitive study that we propose can be operationalized as a study that had findings that were inconsistent with theory or did not replicate previous findings (potential Type II error; where biased designed studies fail to identify relationships that in fact exist). Further, a study was classified as counterintuitive if there was mixed support for the Rorschach variables studied. For example, many research studies in the Mihura et al. meta-analyses examined multiple Rorschach variables (i.e., Hart, 1991). Hart did not find results consistent for the Egocentricity Index (EGOI) but support was found for the other variables examined; however, it was classified as counterintuitive owing to the inconsistent finding for EGOI. The importance of this distinction is, simply stated, if counterintuitive findings occur within a methodologically biased design there is no way to tell if the findings are true findings independent of confounds introduced by the methodology (Type II error; Weiner, 1995b). Specifically, these type of studies (including those with confounds that are not addressed) rarely identify relationships that do not exist (Type I error); rather, counterintuitive findings in Rorschach research often result in a failure to identify relationships that do in fact exist (Type II error). These counterintuitive studies within the validation studies were tallied up and an overall number was calculated.

Results

All 210 articles had some issues in the criteria assessed. When looking at the five criteria globally (IQ/Education level, R, Lambda/F%, interrater reliability, sample size), every article had methodological issues (see Table 1). Four articles only had one methodological issue (1.9%), 17 had two (8.1%), 85 had three (40.5%), 87 had four (41.4%), and 17 had five (8.1%). An example of an article with two problems was the one by Dao and Prevatt (2006). They provided statistics for R, provided an adequate interrater reliability, and had comparison groups greater than 20; however, there was no mention of IQ/Education level or Lambda/F%. An example of an article with five issues was that by Abraham, Mann, Lewis, Coontz, and Lehman (1990). They had three comparison groups of 15 participants, did not provide statistics for R, Lambda/F%, or interrater reliability, and did not provide a range for IQ. The specific questions for the five criteria were also calculated

Table 1. Methodological issues analysis (N = 210)

Methodological issues (n)	Articles (n)	Percentage
0	0	0%
1	4	1.9%
2	17	8.1%
3	85	40.5%
4	87	41.4%
5	17	8.1%

Table 2. Five methodological criteria analysis (N = 210)

Criterion	Articles (n)	Percentage
IQ/Education level		
No M and range	56	26.7%
Missing M or range	118	56.2%
IQ $M < 80$	20	9.5%
Responses (R)		
No M and range	108	51.4%
M reported but no range	65	31.0%
Range reported but no M	2	1.0%
Responses < 14	22	10.5%
Lambda/F%		
No M and range	141	67.1%
$M = L > .99/F\% > .50$	40	19.0%
No range for L/F%	45	21.4%
$M = L > .99/F\% > .50$ & No IQ/Ed. level reported	28	13.3%
Interrater reliability		
None reported	72	34.2%
$< .60$ (κ/ICC) and/or 80% agreement	16	7.6%
Sample size		
< 20 participants	56	26.7%

Note. M = mean; L = Lambda; $F\%$ = percentage of F responses.

(see Table 2). The total calculations show if the answer was *no* to the question asked.

Two independent raters then used the aforementioned operationalizations about application and validation studies and analyzed each of the 210 studies. In total, 106 studies were classified as validation studies; however, there was a

Table 3. Methodological issues in validation studies only (N = 104)

Methodological issues (n)	Articles (n)	Percentage
0	0	0%
1	0	0%
2	12	11.5%
3	34	32.7%
4	50	48.1%
5	8	7.7%

disagreement on three articles. The interrater reliability was measured by kappa ($\kappa = .97$). A third rater resolved the disagreement, and 104 of the 210 studies (49.5%) were classified as validation studies.

Since validation studies are more appropriate for meta-analyses, the 104 studies were analyzed with the same criteria used for all 210 articles (see Table 3 and Table 4). After these analyses, the counterintuitive finding operationalization was used with the 104 validation studies. It was found that 45 studies (43.3%) had counterintuitive findings.

Discussion

Exner and colleagues (1995a; Cunliffe et al., 2012; Gacono et al., 2001; Gacono et al., 2008) provided pertinent caveats for conducting Rorschach research. At this time, there are no set rules for conducting Rorschach research and few have critiqued the points provided by the authors of *Issues and Methods in Rorschach Research* and Gacono et al. (2001). Other researchers have proposed important concepts to consider when conducting Rorschach research (i.e., not using a normative sample as a comparison group); however, the criteria used in this article appear to be the most pertinent to validity and generalizability. Those who research the Rorschach must be aware of these complexities and pitfalls (Exner, 1995a). Failure to heed these cautions produced biased Rorschach studies that led to inaccurate claims about the test (many resulting from Type II error). Most of the researchers did not provide descriptive data for Rorschach samples (Viglione & Exner, 1995). For example, 51.4% did not provide any statistics for R and 67.1% did not provide these data for Lambda/F%. Further, of the 210 articles, 90% had three or more issues, which indicated these articles manifested gaps in their methodology.

A little more than half the articles included in these meta-analyses were application studies (*with* the Rorschach; 50.5%) and this is problematic when

Table 4. Five methodological criteria analysis for validation studies only ($N = 104$)

Criterion	Articles (n)	Percentage
IQ/Education level		
No M and range	27	26.0%
Missing M or range	61	58.7%
IQ $M < 80$	9	8.7%
Responses (R)		
No M and range	58	55.8%
M reported but no range	26	25.0%
Range reported but no M	2	1.9%
Responses < 14	9	8.7%
Lambda/F%		
No M and Range	80	76.9%
$M = L > .99/F\% > .50$	16	15.4%
No range for L/F%	14	13.5%
$M = L > .99/F\% > .50$ & No IQ/Ed. level reported	12	11.5%
Interrater reliability		
None reported	33	31.7%
$< .60$ (κ/ICC) and/or 80% agreement	7	6.7%
Sample size		
< 20 participants	25	24.0%

Note. M = mean; L = Lambda; F% = percentage of F responses.

evaluating the validity of Rorschach variables since this type of study is not meant to validate Rorschach variables. Even more concerning is the fact that these two very different types of research (studies *with* the Rorschach vs. studies *on* the Rorschach) were combined indiscriminately in the Mihura et al. (2013) meta-analyses. Indeed, in application studies, Rorschach variables are typically dependent variables of the research design (e.g., the effects of cognitive remediation on thought disorder in patients with schizophrenia as assessed by the CS WSum6). Treating application studies (*with* the Rorschach) as validation studies (*on* the Rorschach) is the equivalent of confusing dependent and independent variables of research designs.

Since validation studies are more pertinent for a meta-analysis looking to validate Rorschach scores, many of the Rorschach validation studies included in Mihura et al. (2013) meta-analyses did not meet the methodological criteria assessed (90% had three or more problems with the criteria). Failure to meet the five criteria assessed limits the validity and generalizability of the study. If there are problems in a study it may not be advisable to use it in a meta-analysis. Finding a relationship despite poor methodology is more impressive and comes with more weight than failing to find a relationship because of poor methodology. This leaves open the possibility that the relationship exists and can be found with better methods (overcoming Type II error) as poor methodological studies rarely yield Type I error (identifying relationships that do not exist). A more refined analysis of the validation studies was undertaken to determine whether the studies had counterintuitive findings (i.e., were inconsistent with theory and/or previous research). In all, 45 studies had counterintuitive findings (43.3%). Owing to the methodological issues it is unclear if these findings are due to Type II error, the findings are real, an artifact of the methodology, a quirk, or an atypical sample. Moreover, negative results could be attributable to Lambda or EB. That is, a variable could be valid for some purpose among L < 1.00 records; however, it could be invalid among L > 0.99 records, and similarly a variable could be valid for some purpose among introversive but not extratensive records (EB style).

For example, Simon (1989) did not find support of the Isolation Index (one of the variables Mihura et al. suggested had no support) compared with an MMPI scale. However, Simon did not report L/F% and IQ/Education level and included protocols with R < 14 (R = 10). Without even considering the problems when using MMPI scales to validate Rorschach indices, the failure to take into account these criteria, it makes it impossible for the reader to determine whether the lack of correlation between the MMPI scale and the Rorschach index was nothing more than the result of an atypical sample. Hart (1991) looked at the Egocentricity Index (EGOI; another variable identified by Mihura et al. as having poor support) and the results did not support previous findings. However, Hart did not have IQ scores for all the participants, some had IQ < 80, and L/F% and interrater reliability were not reported. Another study examining the EGOI (Brems & Johnson, 1990) also did not find support for the index. However, the participants (inpatient psychiatric patients) had a high Lambda ($M = 1.20$) and IQ/Education level and R statistics were not provided. Ball and colleagues (1991; a study found to contain bias [Dies, 1995a]) found inconsistent findings with the DEPI; however, percent agreement in terms of some Rorschach variables was 60%, much less than the acceptable 80%. Again, these issues from all these studies makes it difficult to generalize the findings.

Although the counterintuitive findings pertain to Type II error, there are problems with Rorschach studies that can lead to Type I error. This would include using a shotgun study (where many statistical analyses are performed), normative samples being used as a comparison group (i.e., Exner, 1995b; Shaffer et al., 1999), or inappropriate statistical comparisons being used (i.e., using parametric statistics like ANOVA rather than a chi-square analysis). Exner (1995b) cautioned that using a normative sample would result in some statistically significant findings by chance and should not be used. This would also be found when using too many comparisons (shotgun studies). Viglione (1995) provided a table of which CS variables are appropriate for parametric analyses (i.e., t test) and which are appropriate for non-parametric (i.e., chi-square) analyses. For example, any content variable is more appropriate for chi-square analyses, while X-% is generally appropriate for parametric analyses. It is often more appropriate with variables such as texture to evaluate this in terms of $T = 0$, $T = 1$, and $T > 1$. This is the case with many Rorschach variables and conducting the correct analysis is essential when examining studies to be included within meta-analyses. Examining the 210 articles in the Mihura et al. meta-analyses, 17 (8.1%) studies met criteria for a shotgun study, 12 (5.7%) had compared their sample with an Exner normative sample, and 70 (33.3%) used inappropriate statistical comparisons (i.e., using parametric statistics like ANOVA rather than a chi-square analysis). Therefore, many studies included in the Mihura et al. (2013) meta-analyses may be problematic because of both Type I and Type II error.

In 1995, Exner stated: "A huge number of published investigations ... are clearly marked by errors in design, implementation, and/or analysis" (Exner, 1995b, p. 3). Further, Viglione and Exner (1995) stated: "A substantial proportion [of Rorschach research] have been marked by flaws" and "all literature cannot be afforded equal weight" (p. 55). Though there have been improvements, this continues to be the case as identified in the analysis. Many of the caveats provided by researchers have not been followed (Dies, 1995a, 1995b; Exner, 1995; Gacono et al., 2001; Ritzler & Exner, 1995; Viglione, 1995; Viglione & Exner, 1995; Weiner, 1995b).

Implications

These results can factor into future Rorschach meta-analytic research. Using more appropriate and methodologically sound studies, the effect sizes may be larger and more power can be given to the findings (overcoming Type I and II errors). Currently, two systems are being used to administer, score, and interpret the Rorschach. The Exner CS and the Rorschach Performance Assessment System (R-PAS; Meyer, Viglione, Mihura, Erard, & Erdberg, 2011). The CS and the R-PAS are two entirely different systems; however, both use the same research foundation. Specifically, "R-PAS variable selection draws heavily on the meta-analyses by Mihura et al. (2013)" (Erard, Meyer, & Viglione, 2014, p. 172) and the "Mihura et al. (2013) results form the foundation for the statements made throughout Chapter 15 [of the R-PAS manual] on Variable Selection and Validity" (p. 172). Therefore, the results would also apply to the R-PAS.

However, the results of this paper should not dampen the spirts of those who use the CS and/or R-PAS or inspire those who have criticized the Rorschach (i.e., Wood and colleagues). It is imperative that researchers who use the

Rorschach produce methodologically sound studies so that any subsequent meta-analytic studies will have more power. Mihura et al. (2013) in a single article took on the challenge to address the validity of each Exner variable. Although critics (Tibon Czopp & Zeligman, 2016; Wood et al., 2015) and to a certain extent this article have commented on it, the Mihura et al. meta-analyses began to address the validity of each Rorschach variable.

Limitations and Future Directions

The five criteria used in the main analyses were gathered from different published Rorschach research. However, there might be other criteria researchers may find important to include in this type of analysis. The five criteria included were expressed by multiple authors; therefore, there appears to be consensus about their importance related to generalizability and validity. Additionally, the concepts expressed in this article may be novel to the reader (*application* vs. *validation studies*; counterintuitive findings). Nevertheless, these concepts are important when examining individual studies included in a meta-analysis. Another limitation is that this analysis only focused on articles referenced in the Mihura et al. (2013) meta-analyses. Therefore, other Rorschach articles not cited may have contained less methodological bias. The Mihura et al. (2013) meta-analytic articles were used because they form the current Rorschach validity research base. Additionally, all articles cited in Mihura et al. were published before 2012. Therefore, current articles may be more methodologically sound. Future studies may examine articles from 2012 to the present with the same analyses (five criteria).

Conclusion

The following can be gleaned from this analysis:

1. Although it was published over 20 years ago, the Exner (1995a) edited book *Issues and Methods in Rorschach Research* is essential reading for any researcher using the Rorschach. The information provided should be followed, which will result in a methodologically sound study (also see Cunliffe et al., 2012; Gacono et al., 2001; Gacono & Gacono, 2008). Improved research designed studies will enhance the validity of the Rorschach.
2. The articles cited in the Mihura et al. (2013) meta-analyses suffered from methodological problems. Therefore, when referring to the meta-analytic

findings, some caution is advised. Further, Mihura et al. (2016) continued a trend to respond to criticism of the meta-analyses from a statistical perspective, rather than acknowledging and addressing issues raised by including poorly designed studies in the meta-analyses.

3. When researchers use the Rorschach in future studies, it is imperative that they understand what influences Rorschach research (i.e., IQ/Educational level), increase interrater reliability, report sample parameters (*M*, *SD*, and frequency for Lambda, R and any variables studied) and include appropriate sample sizes. Without this information the consumer cannot determine whether the statistical procedures in the studies were appropriate and whether the findings can be generalized beyond the sample studied (Gacono & Gacono, 2008; Gacono et al., 2008).

4. There is value in both application and validation studies; however, more validation studies are needed to perform appropriate meta-analyses.

5. It should be noted that some of these methodological issues are not unique to the Rorschach and they appear to be relevant in other psychological measure research (i.e., PAI, MMPI-2).

6. Only articles published before 2012 were reviewed owing to the focus on Mihura et al. (2013). Future research will investigate whether these issues are present in current research (2012 and beyond).

Acknowledgments

Thank you to Dr. Eric Lugo for the Spanish translation of the summary. Opinions expressed in this article are those of the author and do not necessarily represent the opinions of the Federal Bureau of Prisons or the Department of Justice.

References

Abraham, P. P., Mann, T., Lewis, M. G., Coontz, B., & Lehman, M. (1990). The Cognitive Synthesis Test and the Rorschach indicators of internal and external reality in schizophrenic, borderline, and organic/psychotic adolescents. *British Journal of Projective Psychology, 34*, 34–44.

Acklin, M. W., & McDowell, C. I. (1995). Statistical power in Rorschach research. In J. E. Exner (Ed.), *Issues and methods in Rorschach research* (pp. 181–193). Hillsdale, NJ: Erlbaum.

Ball, J. D., Archer, R. P., Gordon, R. A., & French, J. (1991). Rorschach Depression indices with children and adolescents: Concurrent validity findings. *Journal of Personality Assessment, 57*, 465–476. https://doi.org/10.1207/s15327752jpa5703_6

Bannatyne, L., Gacono, C., & Greene, R. (1999). Differential patterns of responding among three groups of chronic, psychotic and forensic outpatients. *Journal of Clinical Psychology, 55*(12), 1553–1565.

Borsboom, D., Mellenbergh, G. J., & van Heerden, J. (2004). The concept of validity. *Psychological Review, 111*(4), 1061–1071.

Brems, C., & Johnson, M. E. (1990). Further exploration of the Egocentricity Index in an inpatient psychiatric population. *Journal of Clinical Psychology, 46*, 675–679. https://doi.org/10.1002/1097-4679(199009)46:5<675::AID-JCLP2270460521 3.0.CO;2-6

Bridges, M., Wilson, J., & Gacono, C. B. (1998). A Rorschach investigation of defensiveness, self-perception, interpersonal relations, and affective states in incarcerated pedophiles. *Journal of Personality Assessment, 70*, 365–385.

Butcher, J. N., Dahlstrom, W. G., Graham, J. R., Tellegen, A., & Kaemmer, B. (1989). *Minnesota Multiphasic Personality Inventory-2 (MMPI-2): Manual for administration. scoring, and interpretation.* Minneapolis, MN: University of Minnesota Press.

Button, K. S., Ioannidis, J. P. A., Mokrysz, C., Nosek, B. A., Flint, J., Robinson, E. S. J., & Munafo, M. R. (2013). Power failure: Why small sample size undermines the reliability of neuroscience. *Nature Reviews Neuroscience, 14*, 365–376.

Cohen, J. (1992). A power primer. *Psychological Bulletin, 112*, 155–159.

Cunliffe, T. B., Gacono, C. B., Meloy, J. R., Smith, J. M., Taylor, E. E., & Landry, D. (2012). Psychopathy and the Rorschach: A response to Wood et al. (2010). *Archives of Assessment Psychology, 2*(1), 1–31.

Dao, T. K., & Prevatt, F. (2006). A psychometric evaluation of the Rorschach Comprehensive System's Perceptual Thinking Index. *Journal of Personality Assessment, 86*, 180–189. https://doi.org/10.1207/s15327752jpa8602_07

Dies, R. (1995a). Conceptual issues in Rorschach research. In J. E. Exner (Ed.), *Issues and methods in Rorschach research* (pp. 25–51). Hillsdale, NJ: Erlbaum.

Dies, R. (1995b). Subject variables in Rorschach research. In J. E. Exner (Ed.), *Issues and methods in Rorschach research* (pp. 99–121). Hillsdale, NJ: Erlbaum.

Erard, R. E., Meyer, G. J., & Viglione, D. J. (2014). Setting the record straight: Comment on Gurley, Piechowski, Sheehan, and Gray (2014) on the admissibility of the Rorschach Performance Assessment System (R-PAS) in court. *Psychological Injury and Law, 7*, 165–177. https://doi.org/10.1007/s12207-014-9195-x

Exner, J. E. (1974). *The Rorschach: A comprehensive system: Vol. 1. Basic foundations* (1st ed.). New York, NY: Wiley.

Exner, J. E. (1986). *The Rorschach: A comprehensive system: Vol. 1. Basic foundations* (2nd ed.). New York, NY: Wiley.

Exner, J. E. (1992). R in Rorschach research: A ghost revisited. *Journal of Personality Assessment, 58*, 245–251.

Exner, J. E. (1993). *The Rorschach: A comprehensive system: Vol. 1. Basic Foundations* (3rd ed.). New York, NY: Wiley.

Exner J. E. (Ed.). (1995a). *Issues and methods in Rorschach research.* Mahwah, NJ: Erlbaum.

Exner, J. E. (1995b). Introduction. In J. E. Exner (Ed.), *Issues and methods in Rorschach research* (pp. 1–24). Mahwah, NJ: Erlbaum.

Exner, J. E. (2003). *The Rorschach: A comprehensive system: Vol. 1. Basic foundations and principles of interpretation* (4th ed.). Hoboken, NJ: Wiley.

Exner, J. E., Kinder, B. N., & Curtis, G. (1995). Reviewing basic design features. In J. E. Exner (Ed.), *Issues and methods in Rorschach research* (pp. 145–158). Mahwah, NJ: Erlbaum.

Gacono, C. B. (1997). Is the Rorschach Aggressive Movement Response enough? *British Journal of Projective Psychology, 42*(2), 5–11.

Gacono, C. B., Evans, F. B., & Viglione, D. J. (2008). Essential issues in the forensic use of the Rorschach. In C. B. Gacono, F. B. Evans, N. Kaser-Boyd, & L. A. Gacono (Eds.), *The handbook of forensic Rorschach assessment* (pp. 3–21). New York, NY: Routledge.

Gacono, C. B., & Meloy, J. R. (1994). *The Rorschach assessment of aggressive and psychopathic personalities*. Hillsdale, NJ: Erlbaum.

Gacono, C. B., Meloy, J. R., & Bridges, M. R. (2000). A Rorschach comparison of psychopaths, sexual homicide perpetrators, and nonviolent pedophiles: Where angels fear to tread. *Journal of Clinical Psychology, 56*, 757–777. https://doi.org/10.1002/(SICI)1097-4679(200006)56:6<757::AID-JCLP6>3.0.CO;2-I

Gacono, L. A., & Gacono, C. B. (2008). Some considerations for the Rorschach assessment of forensic psychiatric outpatients. In C. B. Gacono, F. B. Evans, N. Kaser-Boyd, & L. A. Gacono (Eds.), *The handbook of forensic Rorschach assessment* (pp. 421–444). New York, NY: Routledge/Taylor & Francis Group.

Gacono, C. B., Loving, J. L., & Bodholdt, R. H. (2001). The Rorschach and psychopathy: Toward a more accurate understanding of the research findings. *Journal of Personality Assessment, 77*, 16–38.

Hart, L. R. (1991). The Egocentricity Index as a measure of self-esteem and egocentric personality style for inpatient adolescents. *Perceptual and Motor Skills, 73*, 907–914. https://doi.org/10.2466/PMS.73.7.907-914

Hemphill, J. F. (2003). Interpreting the magnitudes of correlation coefficients. *American Psychologist, 58*, 78–79. https://doi.org/10.1037/0003-066X.58.1.78

Hunter, J. E., & Schmidt, F. L. (2004). *Methods of meta-analysis: Correcting error and bias in research findings* (2nd ed.). Thousand Oaks, CA: Sage.

Kircher, T., Krug, A., Stratmann, M., Ghazi, S., Schales, C., Frauenheim, M., & Grosvald, M. (2014). A rating scale for the assessment of objective and subjective formal Thought and Language Disorder (TALD). *Schizophrenia research, 160*(1), 216–221. https://doi.org/10.1016/j.schres.2014.10.024

Konishi, H. (2003). The lambda in the Rorschach comprehensive system [Original in Japanese]. *Shinrigaku Kenkyu, 73*(6), 502–505.

Mcguire, H., Kinder, B. N., Curtiss, G., & Viglione, D. J. (1995). Some special issues in data analysis. In J. E. Exner (Ed.), *Issues and methods in Rorschach research* (pp. 227–250). Hillsdale, NJ: Erlbaum.

Meyer, G. J. (1992). Response frequency problems in the Rorschach: Clinical and research implications with suggestions for the future. *Journal of Personality Assessment, 58*, 231–244. https://doi.org/10.1207/s15327752jpa5802_2

Meyer, G. J. (1999). Simple procedures to estimate chance agreement and kappa for the interrater reliability of response segments using the Rorschach Comprehensive System. *Journal of Personality Assessment, 72*, 230–255.

Meyer, G. J., Giromini, L., Viglione, D. J., Reese, J. B., & Mihura, J. L. (2015). The association of gender, ethnicity, age, and education with Rorschach scores. *Assessment, 22*, 46–64. https://doi.org/10.1177/1073191114544358

Meyer, G. J., Viglione, D. J., & Exner, J. E. (2001). Superiority of Form% over Lambda for research on the Rorschach Comprehensive System. *Journal of Personality Assessment, 76*, 68–75. https://doi.org/10.1207/S15327752JPA7601_4

Meyer, G. J., Viglione, D. J., Mihura, J. L., Erard, R. E., & Erdberg, P. (2011). *Rorschach performance assessment system: Administration, coding, interpretation, and technical manual*. Toledo, OH: Rorschach Performance Assessment System.

Mihura, J. L., Meyer, G. J., Dumitrascu, N., & Bombel, G. (2013). The validity of individual Rorschach variables: Systematic reviews and meta-analyses of the comprehensive system. *Psychological Bulletin, 139*, 548–605. https://doi.org/10.1037/a0029406

Mihura, J. L., Meyer, G. J., Bombel, G., & Dumitrascu, N. (2015). Standards, accuracy, and questions of bias in Rorschach meta-analyses: Reply to Wood, Garb, Nezworski, Lilienfeld, and Duke (2015). *Psychological Bulletin, 141*, 250–260. https://doi.org/10.1037/a0038445

Mihura, J. L., Meyer, G. J., Bombel, G., & Dumitrascu, N. (2016). On conducting construct validity meta-analyses for the Rorschach: A reply to Tibon Czopp and Zeligman (2016). *Journal of Personality Assessment, 98*(4), 343–350. https://doi.org/10.1080/00223891.2016.1158182

Millon, T., Grossman, S., & Millon, C. (2015). *Millon Clinical Multiaxial Inventory-IV manual*. Minneapolis, MN: Pearson.

Morey, L. C. (1991). *Personality Assessment Inventory manual*. Odessa, FL: Psychological Assessment Resources.

Ritzler, B. A., & Exner, J. E. (1995). Special issues in subject selection and design. In J. E. Exner (Ed.), *Issues and methods in Rorschach research* (pp. 123–143). Hillsdale, NJ: Erlbaum.

Sánchez-Meca, J., & Marín-Martínez, F. (2010). Meta-analysis in psychological research. *International Journal of Psychological Research, 3*(1), 151–163.

Shaffer, T. W., Erdberg, P., & Haroian, J. (1999). Current nonpatient data for the Rorschach, WAIS-R, and MMPI-2. *Journal of Personality Assessment, 73*(2), 305–316.

Simon, M. J. (1989). Comparison of the Rorschach Comprehensive System's Isolation Index and MMPI Social Introversion score. *Psychological Reports, 65*, 499–502. https://doi.org/10.2466/pr0.1989.65.2.499

Tibon Czopp, S., & Zeligman, R. (2016). The Rorschach Comprehensive System (CS) psychometric validity of individual variables. *Journal of Personality Assessment, 98*(4), 335–342. https://doi.org/ 10.1080/00223891.2015.1131162

Viglione, D. J. (1995). Basic considerations regarding data analysis. In J. E. Exner (Ed.), *Issues and methods in Rorschach research* (pp. 195–226). Hillsdale, NJ: Erlbaum.

Viglione, D. J. (1999). A review of recent research addressing the utility of the Rorschach. *Psychological Assessment, 11*(3), 251–265.

Viglione, D. J., & Exner, J. E. (1995). Formulating issues in Rorschach research. In J. E. Exner (Ed.), *Issues and methods in Rorschach research* (pp. 53–71). Hillsdale, NJ: Erlbaum.

Viglione, D. J., & Meyer, G. J. (2008). An overview of psychometrics for forensic practice. In C. B. Gacono, F. B. Evans, N. Kaser-Boyd, & L. A. Gacono (Eds.), *The handbook of forensic Rorschach assessment* (pp. 21–54). New York, NY: Routledge.

Weiner, I. B. (1966). *Psychodiagnostics in schizophrenia*. New York, NY: Wiley.

Weiner, I. B. (1995a). Methodological considerations in Rorschach research. *Psychological Assessment, 7*(3), 330–337.

Weiner, I. B. (1995b). Variable selection in Rorschach research. In J. E. Exner (Ed.), *Issues and methods in Rorschach research* (pp. 73–97). Hillsdale, NJ: Erlbaum.

Weiner, I. B. (2003). *Principles of Rorschach interpretation* (2nd ed.). Mahwah, NJ: Erlbaum.

Wood, J. M., Garb, H. N., Nezworski, M. T., Lilienfeld, S. O., & Duke, M. C. (2015). A second look at the validity of widely used Rorschach indices: Comment on Mihura, Meyer, Dumitrascu, and Bombel (2013). *Psychological Bulletin, 141*, 236–249. https://doi.org/10.1037/a0036005

Wood, J. M., Lilienfeld, S. O., Nezworski, M. T., Garb, H. N., Holloway Allen, K., & Wildermuth, J. L. (2010). Validity of Rorschach inkblot scores for discriminating psychopaths from nonpsychopaths in forensic populations: A meta-analysis. *Psychological Assessment, 22*(2), 336–349. https://doi.org/10.1037/a0018998

Wood, J. M., Nezworski, M. T., & Stejskal, W. J. (1996). The Comprehensive System for the Rorschach: A critical examination. *Psychological Science, 7*, 3–10. https://doi.org/10.1111/j.1467-9280.1996.tb00658.x

Zillmer, E. A., & Vuz, J. K. (1995). Factor analysis with Rorschach data. In J. E. Exner (Ed.), *Issues and methods in Rorschach research* (pp. 251–306). Hillsdale, NJ: Erlbaum.

Received December 3, 2016
Revision received October 22, 2017
Accepted February 5, 2018
Published online November 9, 2018

Jason M. Smith
FCC Hazelton
Bruceton Mills, WV
USA
jmsmithpsyd@gmail.com

Summary

Exner's *Issues and Methods in Rorschach Research* (1995a) provided a standard of care for conducting Rorschach research; however, the extent to which studies have followed these guidelines has not been examined. Similarly, meta-analytic approaches have been used to comment on the validity of Comprehensive System (CS) variables without an evaluation as to the extent the individual studies have conformed to proposed methodological criteria (Exner, 1995a; Gacono, Loving, & Bodholdt, 2001). In this article, the 210 studies cited in recent Mihura, Meyer, Dumitrascu, and Bombel (2013) meta-analyses were examined. Individual studies were analyzed for: research *on the Rorschach* versus research *with the Rorschach* and whether they met the threshold of validity/generalizability related to specific Rorschach criteria. These criteria were: (1) IQ/Education Level; (2) Responses; (3) Lambda; (4) interrater reliability; and (5) sample size. Out of 210, 104 (49.5%) studies focused on research *on the Rorschach* and none met all five Rorschach criteria assessed. Further, 90% of the studies examined had three or more issues related to the above criteria. Therefore, the Exner (1995a) edited book *Issues and Methods in Rorschach Research* is essential reading for any researcher using the Rorschach. When researchers use the Rorschach in future studies, it is imperative that they understand what influences Rorschach research (i.e., IQ/Education level), increase interrater reliability, use appropriate statistics, report sample parameters (M, SD, and frequency for Lambda/R and any variables studied), and include appropriate sample sizes. Without this information the consumer cannot determine whether the statistical procedures in the studies were appropriate and whether the findings can be generalized beyond the sample studied. Further, there is value in both application and validation studies; however, more validation studies are needed to perform appropriate meta-analyses. The results of this paper should not dampen the spirts of those who use the CS and/or R-PAS or inspire those who have criticized the Rorschach (i.e., Wood and colleagues). It is imperative that researchers who use the Rorschach produce methodologically sound studies so that any subsequent meta-analytic studies will have more power.

Résumé

L'ouvrage *Issues and Methods in Rorschach Research* (Exner, 1995a) présente des recommandations concernant les standards de la recherche Rorschach; cependant, la mesure dans laquelle les recherches publiées ont suivi ces lignes directrices n'a pas été examinée. De même, des approches méta-analytiques ont permis d'évaluer la validité des variables du Système Intégré, mais sans prise en compte de la qualité méthodologique des études examinées au regard des standards proposés par Exner, 1995a; puis Gacono, Loving & Bodholdt (2001). Dans cet article, les 210 études citées dans les dernières méta-analyses de Mihura, Meyer, Dumitrascu et Bombel (2013) ont été examinées selon les critères suivants : recherche de validation (sur le Rorschach) vs recherche d'application (avec Rorschach) d'une part et d'autre part les critères suivants : (1) IQ / niveau d'éducation; (2) Nombre de Réponses; (3) Lambda; (4) fiabilité inter-évaluateur; et (5) Taille de l'échantillon. Sur 210, 104 (49,5%) des études étaient des études de validation à proprement parler et aucune ne remplissait l'ensemble des critères méthodologiques évalués. En outre, 90% des études examinées présentait au moins trois problèmes méthodologiques. Par conséquent, le livre *Issues and Methods in Rorschach Research* (Exner, 1995a) est une lecture essentielle pour tout chercheur utilisant le Rorschach. A l'avenir, il est impératif que les chercheurs comprennent les facteurs susceptibles d'influencer la recherche sur le Rorschach : QI, fiabilité inter-évaluateur, utilisation des statistiques appropriées, présentation détaillée des paramètres de l'échantillon (*M*, *SD* et fréquence pour Lambda / R et toutes les variables étudiées) et tailles d'échantillon appropriées. Sans ces informations, le consommateur ne peut pas déterminer si les procédures statistiques employées dans une étude étaient appropriées et si les résultats peuvent être généralisés au-delà de l'échantillon étudié. En outre, si les études d'application et de validation présentent chacune leut intérêt; il semble nécessaire d'entreprendre de nouvelles études de validation pour effectuer des méta-analyses appropriées. Les résultats de cet article ne devraient pas décourager ceux qui utilisent le CS et / ou le R-PAS ou encourager ceux qui ont critiqué le Rorschach (c'est-à-dire Wood et ses collègues). Il est impératif que les chercheurs qui utilisent le Rorschach produisent des études solides sur le plan méthodologique ce qui permettra d'augmenter la puissance de méta-analyses ultérieures.

Resumen

Exner (1995a) *Issues and Methods in Rorschach Research* proporcionó un estándar de precaución para la realización de la investigación de Rorschach. Sin embargo, no se ha examinado hasta qué punto los estudios han seguido estas pautas. Del mismo modo, los enfoques meta-analíticos se han utilizado para comentar la validez de las variables de CS sin una evaluación que incluya los estudios individuales ajustado a los criterios metodológicos propuestos (Exner, 1995a; Gacono, Loving, & Bodholdt, 2001). En este artículo se examinaron los 210 estudios citados en los recientes meta-análisis de Mihura, Meyer, Dumitrascu y Bombel (2013). Se analizaron los estudios individuales para: investigación *sobre el Rorschach* versus investigación *con el Rorschach* y si cumplían el umbral de validez / generalización relacionado con los criterios específicos de Rorschach. Estos criterios fueron 1) CI / Nivel de educación; 2) Respuestas; 3) Lambda; 4) Confiabilidad entre evaluadores; y 5) Tamaño de muestra. De 210, 104 (49.5%) estudios se enfocaron en la investigación del Rorschach y ninguno cumplió con los cinco criterios de Rorschach evaluados. Además, el 90% de los estudios examinados tenían tres o más problemas relacionados con los criterios mencionados anteriores. Por lo tanto, el libro editado de Exner (1995a) *Issues and Methods in Rorschach Research* es una lectura esencial para cualquier investigador que use el Rorschach. Cuando los investigadores utilicen el Rorschach en estudios futuros, es imperativo que entiendan qué influencia tiene la investigación de Rorschach (e.g. CI), aumento de la confiabilidad entre evaluadores, uso de estadísticas apropiadas, información de los parámetros de la muestra (M, DE, y frecuencia para Lambda / R y cualquier variable estudiada) e incluye tamaños de muestra apropiados. Sin esta información, el consumidor no puede determinar si los procedimientos estadísticos de los estudios fueron apropiados y si los resultados pueden generalizarse más allá de la muestra estudiada. Además, hay validez en los estudios de aplicación y validación; sin embargo, se necesitan más estudios de validez para realizar los meta-análisis apropiados. Los resultados de este documento no deben desalentar a los espíritus de quienes usan el CS y / o R-PAS o inspirar a aquellos que han criticado el Rorschach (e.g. Wood y sus colegas). Es imperativo que los investigadores que usan el Rorschach produzcan estudios metodológicamente sólidos para que cualquier estudio meta-analítico posterior tenga más poder.

要約

Exner (1995a) のロールシャッハ研究の問題と方法の再検討

　Exner (1995a) の"ロールシャッハ研究の問題と方法"はロールシャッハ研究をおこなう際に配慮すべき基準を提供したが、どの程度の研究がこのガイドラインに従って実行されたのかについては検討されてきてはいない。同様に、ロールシャッハ包括システムの変数の妥当性についてコメントするのにメタ分析アプローチが用いられてきているが、個々の研究が提唱された方法論的な基準 (Exner, 1995; Gacono, Bodholdt, & Loving, 2001) に対してどの程度適合しているかについての評価はされていない。本論文では近年、Mihura, Meyer, Dumitrascu, and Bombel (2013)に引用された210の研究のメタ分析をおこなった。個々の研究は次のように分析された：ロールシャッハの研究　対　ロールシャッハを用いての研究、これらの研究は特定のロールシャッハの基準に関係する妥当性／一般性に合致しているかどうか。これらの基準は次のようなものである。(1) IQ／教育レベル、(2) 反応数、(3) ラムダ、(4) 評定者間の信頼性、(5) サンプルサイズ。210のうち、104 (49.5％) はロールシャッハの研究に焦点を当てたものであり、これらの研究にロールシャッハの5つの基準をすべて満たしたものはなかった。さらに90％の研究がこれらの基準に関連する3つかそれ以上の問題を有していることが明らかになった。ゆえに、Exner (1995)が編集したロールシャッハの問題と方法はロールシャッハを用いる研究者にとっての必須の書籍であると言える。研究者が将来の研究でロールシャッハをもちいようとする場合、何がロールシャッハの研究に影響を与え (換言すればIQ)、評定者間の信頼性を高めるかを理解し、適切な統計手法を使い、標本のパラメータ (M、SD、ラムダ／Rの頻度や、他の分析されている変数) を示し、適切なサンプルサイズを含むことが必然的になる。これらの情報なしでは消費者は、この研究の統計的手続きが適切かどうか、見出されたことは研究のサンプルを超えて一般化できるかどうかを決めることはできない。さらに、応用研究や妥当性の研究は有用であるが、さらに妥当性の研究は適切なメタ分析を実行する必要がある。本研究の結果は包括システム／R-PASを使用するものの熱意を低下させ、ロールシャッハを批判するもの (Woodやその同僚) を活気づけるものではない。ロールシャッハを用いる研究者は方法論的に健全な研究を生み出すことが必然であり、必然的にメタ分析研究は有力になるであろう。

Book Review

Handbook of Gender and Sexuality in Psychological Assessment

Marianne Nygren

Virginia M. Brabender
Joni L. Mihura (2016)
Handbook of Gender and Sexuality in Psychological Assessment
New York, NY: Routledge
ISBN (hardcover) 978-1-138-782-4-4

Although it is inevitable that assessors and clients think about each other in gender-based terms, this is not always given enough attention in psychological assessments. The present book elucidates the influence of sex, gender, and gender identity on various aspects of the assessment process. The book is valuable and informative for students and early career clinicians working with psychological assessment, but perhaps even more so for midcareer and senior assessors who did not get sufficient training and supervision related to sex and gender in their education. The book is also informative for the reader interested in research.

The necessity of a multimethod approach that also considers all the facets of identity and their consequences for patients runs as the main thread through all the contributions in the book and is well elucidated in the case illustrations. The reader wanting to learn more about the pros and cons of different methods of assessment of socially charged aspects of gender and sex will find rich material in this book. However, many of the aspects explained are relevant for the assessment of persons belonging to minority groups and not only relevant to sex and gender aspects, although these are the focus of the book.

The book is organized in six sections, each with contributions from authorities in their respective fields. These parts are titled:

- Introductory Chapters
- Assessment Tools
- Personality, Psychopathology, and Gender-Based Issues

- Case Illustrations of Gender-Based Issues
- Gender, Sexual Orientation, and Development Status
- Looking Forward

The first section constitutes a good platform for the further reading of the book. Central concepts concerning sexual orientation and gender characteristics and their interaction are defined and the need for more awareness of gender and sexuality in clinical assessment and in assessment research is clarified.

In a short review like this one it is not possible to comment on all the contributions to the book. However, I will comment on some aspects that are focused on by many of the authors.

The vulnerability related to sexual minority and the importance of treating patients from these groups with respect and genuine knowledge and interest are covered in several chapters. Studies of relevant literature (e.g., the different chapters of this handbook) and supervision are important in psychological assessors' education and further training. Moreover, the importance of the assessors' awareness of their own sex, gender, and sexuality identities is emphasized by several of the authors.

Different assessment methods have different pros and cons, and this is well elucidated in the second part of the book. The importance of the assessor's consideration of normative and validation data is pointed out in most chapters.

The influence and justification of gendered norms in cognitive assessment and in self-report personality measures are presented and discussed in an informative way. The problem with face validity, which is most evident in self-report measures where self-presenting confounds may influence the results and be responsible for reported gender differences, is discussed by several authors. Individuals can be more willing to acknowledge behaviors and thoughts they regard consistent with social gender role expectations. Patients may even actively conceal their sexual identity to avoid rejection. It is important for the assessor to be aware of this and to be curious about the patient's history and social and cultural background. Although no assessment method is independent of the patient's efforts to stand out in a favorable light, performance-based instruments are less influenced by such manipulations than other psychological assessment methods. Again, one is reminded of the necessity to use a multimethod assessment approach and of the importance of focusing on meaningful divergences between tests engaging different psychological processes.

In almost all chapters on assessment methods the problem with assessor effects is addressed. All psychological assessments are, directly or indirectly, interpersonal settings and consequently influenced by the identities of both patient and assessor. Assessor effects is always a factor to take into consideration in psychological assessment. They are of vital importance both as a possible source of error but also as an important source of information, and the assessor needs to be observant of how gender influences the collaborative assessment process. Even in the most standardized assessment situations, the treatment the patient experiences from the assessor is of importance, for example, gender role stereotypes may even influence who is referred for cognitive assessment.

To sum up, this handbook presents information from many different angles. Of course, it can be read from cover to cover, but most readers will probably start with the chapters treating aspects of psychological assessment that are closest to their own work and interest. Most of the subjects discussed are applicable in different cultures, although, as the editors mention, the book is mostly focused on US literature.

The book is a valuable and sometimes even entertaining contribution to a field that needs more attention in psychological assessment.

Reviewer: Marianne Nygren, Private Practice, Stockholm, Sweden, marianne_nygren@telia.com, https://doi.org/10.1027/1192-5604/a000105

Instructions to Authors

Rorschachiana is the scientific publication of the International Society for the Rorschach. The journal is interested in advancing theory and clinical applications of the Rorschach and other projective techniques, and research work that can enhance and promote projective methods.

Rorschachiana **publishes the following types of articles:** Original Articles, Research Articles, and Case Studies.

Manuscript Submission: Manuscripts should be submitted online at http://www.editorialmanager.com/ror
Detailed instructions to authors are provided at **http://www.hogrefe.com/j/rorschachiana/**

Copyright Agreement: By submitting an article, the author confirms and guarantees on behalf of him-/herself and any coauthors that he or she holds all copyright in and titles to the submitted contribution, including any figures, photographs, line drawings, plans, maps, sketches and tables, and that the article and its contents do not infringe in any way on the rights of third parties. The author indemnifies and holds harmless the publisher from any third-party claims. The author agrees, upon acceptance of the article for publication, to transfer to the publisher on behalf of him-/herself and any coauthors the exclusive right to reproduce and distribute the article and its contents, both physically and in nonphysical, electronic, and other form, in the journal to which it has been submitted and in other independent publications, with no limits on the number of copies or on the form or the extent of the distribution. These rights are transferred for the duration of copyright as defined by international law. Furthermore, the author transfers to the publisher the following exclusive rights to the article and its contents:

1. The rights to produce advance copies, reprints, or offprints of the article, in full or in part, to undertake or allow translations into other languages, to distribute other forms or modified versions of the article, and to produce and distribute summaries or abstracts.
2. The rights to microfilm and microfiche editions or similar, to the use of the article and its contents in videotext, teletext, and similar systems, to recordings or reproduction using other media, digital or analog, including electronic, magnetic, and optical media, and in multimedia form, as well as for public broadcasting in radio, television, or other forms of broadcast.
3. The rights to store the article and its content in machine-readable or electronic form on all media (such as computer disks, compact disks, magnetic tape), to store the article and its contents in online databases belonging to the publisher or third parties for viewing or downloading by third parties, and to present or reproduce the article or its contents on visual display screens, monitors, and similar devices, either directly or via data transmission.
4. The rights to reproduce and distribute the article and its contents by all other means, including photomechanical and similar processes (such as photocopying or facsimile), and as part of so-called document delivery services.
5. The right to transfer any or all rights mentioned in this agreement, as well as rights retained by the relevant copyright clearing centers, including royalty rights to third parties.

Online Rights for Journal Articles: Guidelines on authors' rights to archive electronic version of their manuscripts online are given in the document "Guidelines on sharing and use of articles in Hogrefe journals" on the journal's web page at www.hogrefe.com/j/rorschachiana

September 2016